The invisible
sense of
the heart

Karen Woodley

Karen is a qualified Dance Movement Psychotherapist whose approach is Person-Centred and humanistic, with a somatic, body based and transpersonal orientation. She trained at Masters level and is registered with the Association for Dance Movement Psychotherapy (ADMP) UK.

Having completed an Advanced Diploma in Counselling Supervision (level 7), accredited by the National Counselling Society (NCS), she hopes to build a solid supervision practice for all those working in the caring professions and is available if you would like to enquire.

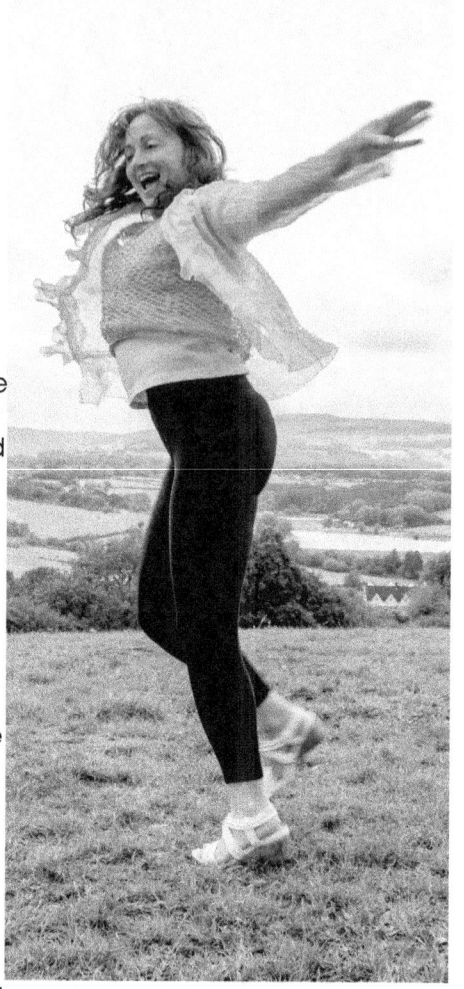

Karen has worked with children, adolescents and adults with learning disabilities, autism and other complex needs for thirty years, starting off as a Montessori Teacher since 1993 where her teaching groups were based around movements and dances from the beginning! She has also worked as a Creative Movement Facilitator in many schools and colleges across the UK and France.

Her training in Biodanza and having been the Director of the Biodanza School Wales years ago where she tutored and supervised new teachers as well as pioneered the technique in the UK led her to her studies as a Movement Psychotherapist. She has specialities in Children, The Four Elements, The Archetypes, The Inner Angels, the Minotaur Project amongst many others.

Karen worked for many years for the Touch Trust Charity in Cardiff Bay as a Senior Session Leader and Training Development Coordinator where she trained and mentored many leaders across Wales. Responsible for the quality of the programme and its delivery to the disabled community, she was the inspiration behind the 'Time for me' project for carers that runs today.

She is the author of 'Tango Therapy – (an Approach to)', 'The Archetypes' DVD and has written many articles such as 'Touch Trust, Health and Well-being through Movement for PMLD link as well as 'Therapy for those with learning disabilities' for the Carers Network magazine.

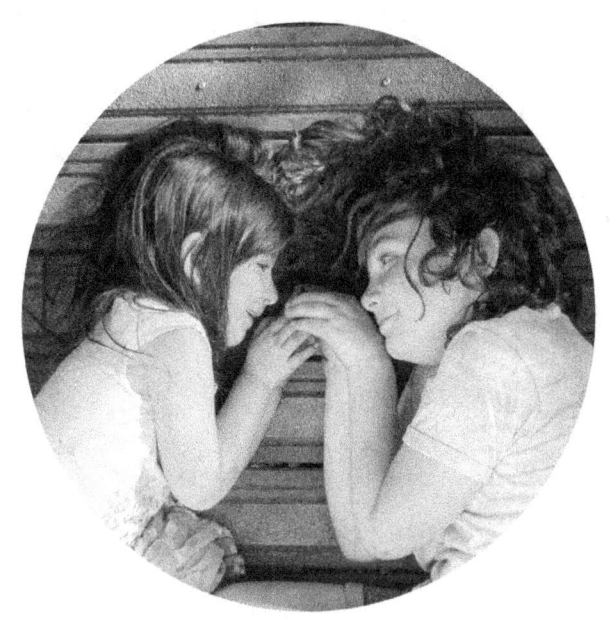

The invisible sense of the heart

"A self-care book for carers with simple ideas for working with children with additional needs"

by Karen Woodley
Dance Movement Psychotherapist – RDMP

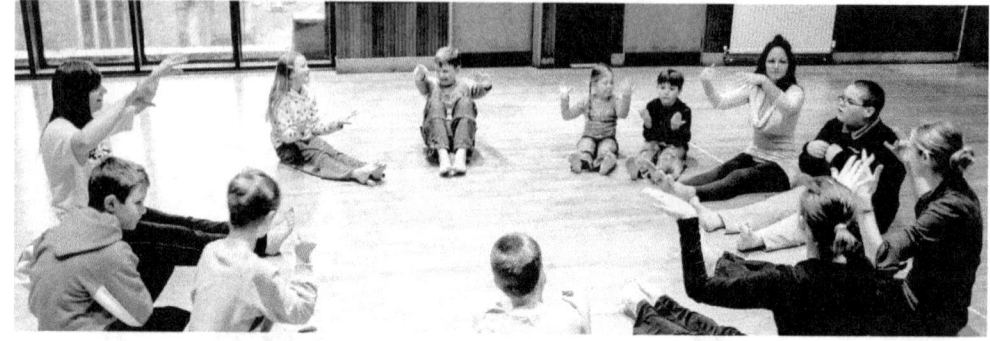

The invisible sense of the heart

"A self-care book for carers with simple ideas for working with children with additional needs"

By Karen Woodley
www.karenwoodley.com / www.danceyourfeelings.com

Photography by Martin Sotelano unless otherwise stated.
www.sotelano.co.uk

This edition first published in 2018 by
Tango Creations
Wales, United Kingdom
www.tangocreations.co.uk
info@tangocreations.co.uk

ISBN 978-0-244-10678-2
Content ID: 23238386

Printed by Lulu

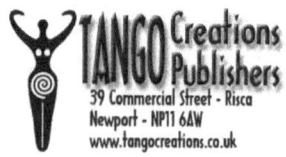

TANGO Creations Publishers
39 Commercial Street - Risca
Newport - NP11 6AW
www.tangocreations.co.uk

*For those who have the courage
to let the fire of their hearts
guide them.*

*Dedicated to my son Llawdden
and my daughter Crisiant.
The lights in my life*

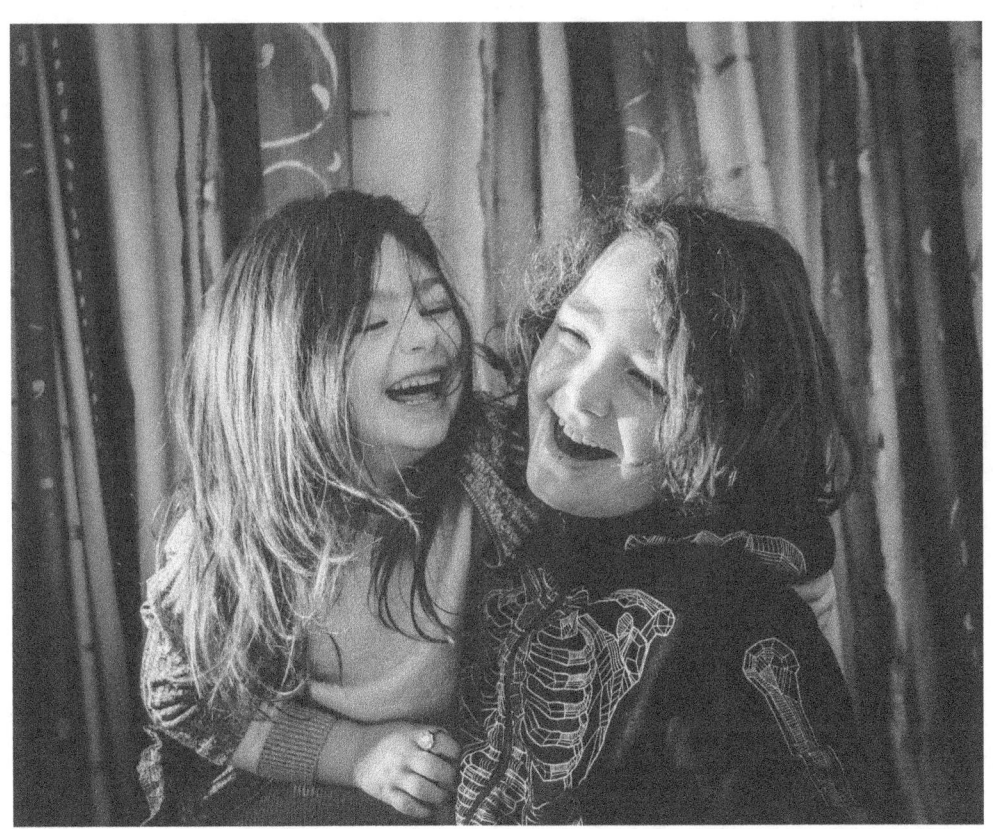

Contents

Introduction: 9

Different ways of learning and learning disabilities   11

• Learning Disabilities   11

• PMLD   12

• ADHD   13

• Dyspraxia   13

• The sixth sence   13

• The learning-disabled child: 14

• Stress and the parent   15

• Time of the diagnosis   16

• Mirror Neurons   17

• Containing and Safety   17

Neuroscience, Dance and Autism

Neuroscience Research and Dance Movement Psychotherapy   19

'Connecting with your body and spirit is an essential part of self-care'   21

• Love flow   21

• Affection   23

• Mirroring   24

• Presence   26

• Honesty   27

The Language of Touch   29

• The Effects of Contact and touch at Organic and Existential level   29

• Touch and Movement   30

• We learn about the world through our bodies   32

Body Movement   34

• Your Spirit   39

• Animal Dances   40

• Just dance!   43

• Give your light   44

Putting life in the centre and Ideas for adding a little love at home   48

Some exercises and ideas that can help to awaken the beautiful inner light of your heart   49

- Connection   49
- A communication key   51
- Affection   54

Colourful Notes   61

- Mimi and her family   61
- George and family   62
- Glenda and mum   62

The Power of the heart   63

Healing Hands and Sensory Movement training programme   65

- 'Enlighten the lives of those you touch'   65

Closing words   67

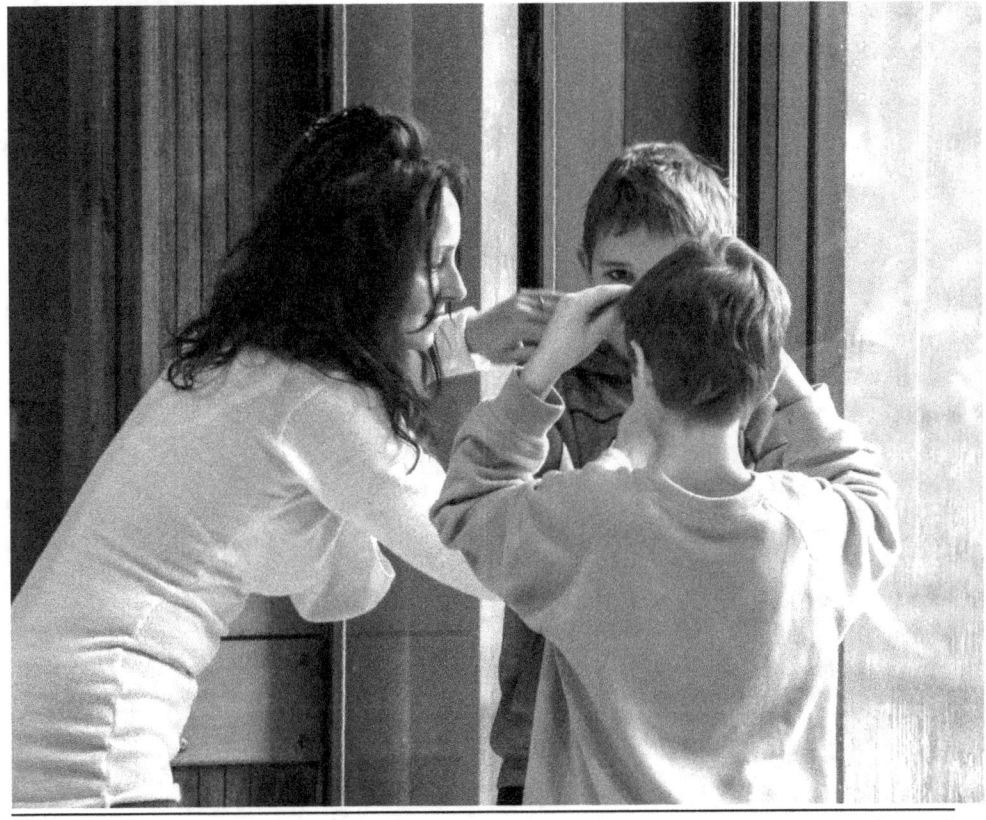

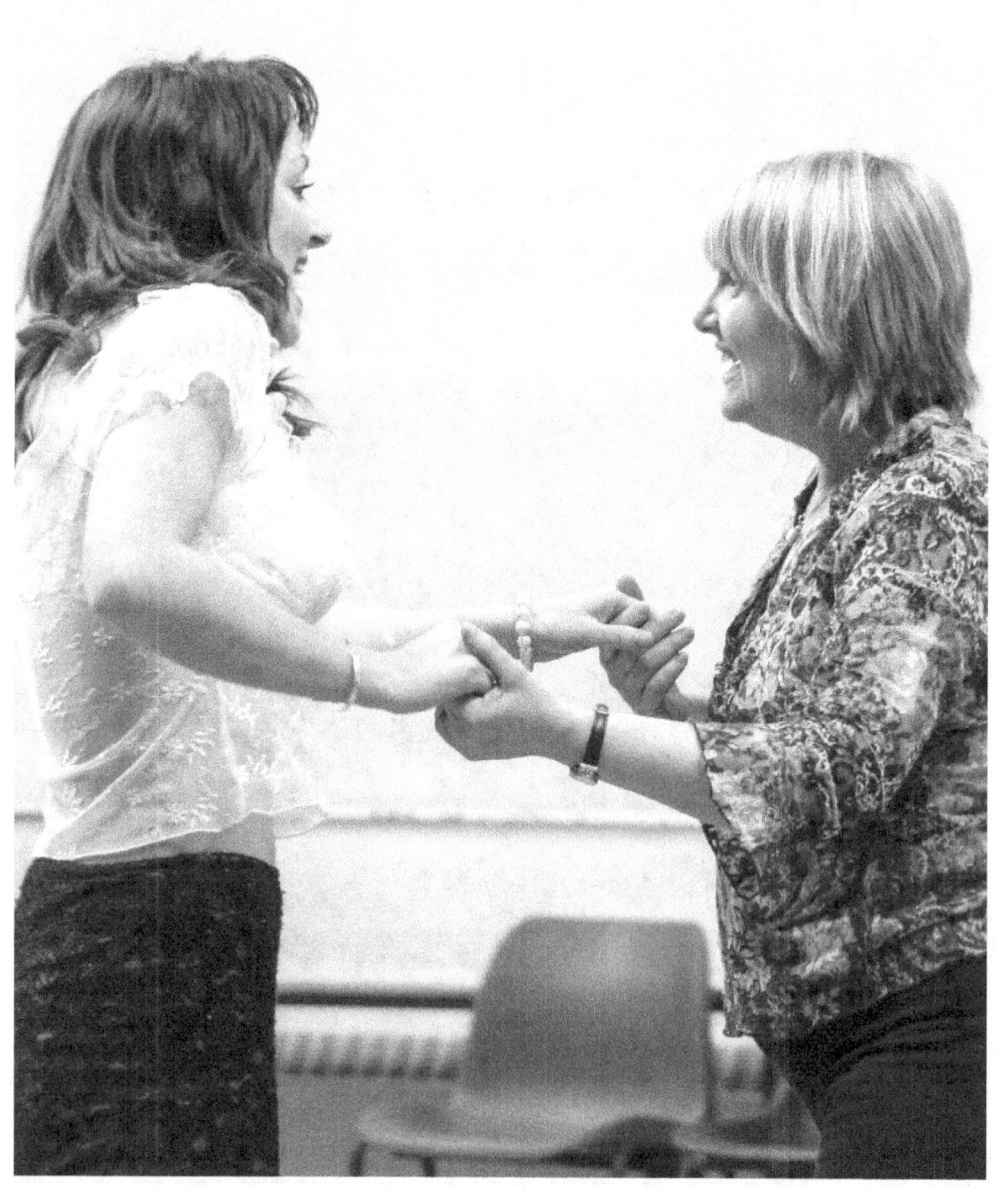

Introduction:

As a carer you have a deeply important job and one that must not go by unnoticed. Taking care of others is the most important job you can do and often goes unnoticed in a culture where doing and competing are more admirable than being and sharing. I know from my own experience that when your work directly involves caring for the emotional, physical and overall well-being of another or others that it is imperative to manage your own vibrant health and physical, emotional and spiritual well-being.

I put this book together as a result of my own encounters as a therapist with children and adults who have learning disabilities as well as my understanding of the great commitment that carers have toward others. I have seen many people give up on themselves and their dreams because they are too exhausted and without simple resources for a little help. Although this booklet is focused on children with additional learning needs it can be applied to anybody in a role where caring for another is your job.

This book offers ideas that you can use to enhance your experience together, help your child / friend to grow with confidence, safety and love. You can start to see yourself as a guardian angel, someone who tends to and guides. So, the idea behind this is also to invite you to see with the eyes of someone whose job it is to 'hold and nurture' and not just to be concerned with personal care issues and functional duties, though these are necessary.

> Three steps:
> 1. be honest with yourself
> 2. be gentle and kind with yourself
> 3. listen with your body

At the end of the day we all at the deepest level have needs, our feelings let us know this through our body. If we ignore our own needs for connection, well-being, honesty and meaning for example then we are repressing our life energy. The same goes for our feelings. If we ignore our feelings of tenderness, curiosity, anger or pain just to pick a few, then we will somehow or another become disconnected from ourselves and others, sick with holding everything in!

I have witnessed this, I have experienced this and I believe that through simple daily practices you can change your life around. Here, exercises and meditations are given that can be explored as part of a self-care practice. Acknowledging that you have needs yourself and that somehow in order to really be the best help to someone else you need to be the best carer to yourself is the first and hardest step of this book.

Even if you only have 5/10mins each day I urge you to begin to take time and focus in on you. I guarantee that you will slowly begin to feel lighter, gentler and not so alone or tired or whatever it is that you feel and experience day to day. Things like taking yourself out for a walk to absorb nature, indulging in weekly massages; not making commitments out of guilt for example. It is not always easy as we have been educated and conditioned to not listen to and trust our inner feelings, our bodily wisdom.

Here I am sharing with you some ways to help you to be more inwardly aware and ways that will help you from this inner awareness to find resources that will make your life and that of your client or companion more pleasurable and easy.

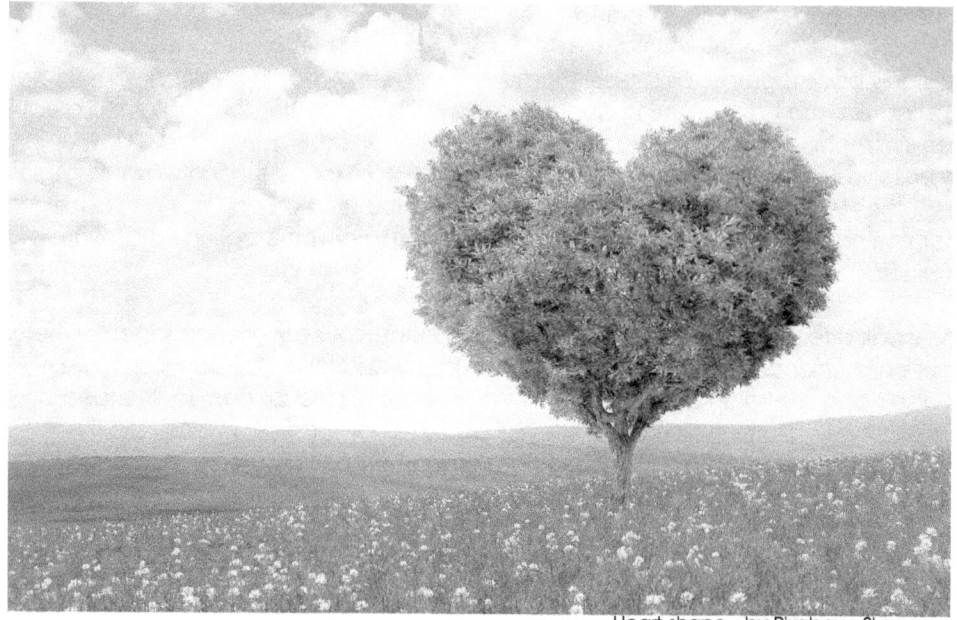

Heart-shape - by Pixabay - Skeeze

Understand that we are all healers and we just need to trust the humanity that flows from our hearts if we allow it! To know that the embryo that makes the heart is the same one that makes the hands so reaching out to another with hands full of tenderness, that come from your heart is the most simplest and most powerful thing you can do.

Understand also that this book is not about meditating and sitting still in a way to clear your mind and breathe through one nostril, keep your back straight and make sure your index finger and thumb are curled together on top of your knees! NO. The idea is to move into a body based experience and flow with yourself and the life around you. Being gentle and kind with yourself is the second step.
The invitation of this book is to read it easy with your body and not your mind. This means noticing as you read, the sensations in your body, the fleeting thoughts and feelings that flow in and out of your awareness. This is the third step which was borne out of my research dissertation that showed that only through an embodied awareness are we able to flow with feeling, aliveness, memory, imagination, dreaming, play and be a force of change in the world.

PART ONE

Different ways of learning and learning disabilities

*"What counts in life is not the mere fact that we have lived.
It is what difference we have made to the lives of others
that will determine the significance of the life we lead"*

Mandela

Children learn in different ways and one of the big mistakes of our "Modern Educational System "(a most basic explanation), is that it is predominantly aimed towards the child who learns in a "logical" manner. A developmental psychologist (Howard Gardner, 1993) argues that the human brain has a wide range of cognitive abilities. He talks about there being nine intelligences that if we can be aware of them can be the pathway into the child's education.

There are ways of being with that can empower the child in beautiful ways and at the same time empower yourself as the parent, teacher or support worker and carer.

Learning Disabilities

There are different types of learning disabilities. Some are mild where the person has no problems making friends and, in social situations only, needs help with things like filling out forms etc. The more severe learning disability is where the person needs more caring support with movement, with communication and with personal care. The child who presents with difficulties in completing schoolwork may not have a cognitive impairment or disability at all rather an emotional need that if not addressed can become a disability.

A theory is that the learning disabilities stem from disturbances that may begin before birth, so in the womb. Also, possibly genetic disposition, alcohol, substance abuse, problems in pregnancy, environmental toxins, central nervous system infections or severe head trauma.

According to Mencap there are different types which can be mild, moderate or severe and in all cases it is lifelong.It is difficult to diagnose a mild form as the child / adult will often mix well and deal well with everyday things.

An affective neuroscientist Damasio says that it is through our emotional feeling system that we know and understand others and the world around us and Since some children with disabilities remain on the pre-verbal level, non-verbal techniques such as dance therapy are the best as they reach and activate the child. Revitalise them through the body, re-establishing a sense of trust in oneself and others; aid in re-socialisation and provides an outlet for discharge of tension, frustration and hostility.

Moreover, the capacity for learning, memory and for perception is deeply conditioned by the affection. The whole process of intelligent adaptation to the environment and ones construction of the world is organised around the first, primal experiences of the affective relationship.

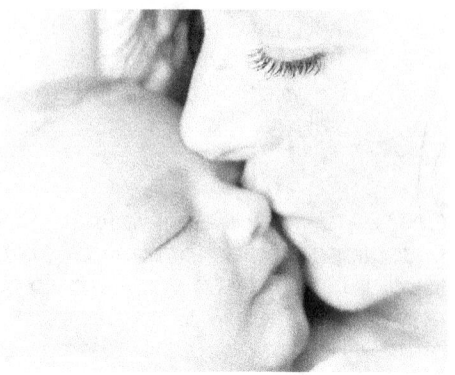

The idea is to keep alive the movement impulse (Bartenieff) the root of all development in working with the emotional well-being in children as well as replace intellectualized movement which tends to encourage dissociation of mind and body with harmony and well-being through breathing, muscular fluctuation and feeling (Bartenieff)

Through a process of focusing on the care/affection and love of the child in the learning process, on the feeling states and stimulation of self-esteem and social skills this process can address:

- Conflictive behaviours
- Lack of concentration
- The expression of aggression
- Expansion and expression of emotional states

In applying the Healing Hands and Sensory Movement training programme the concerns are with the behaviour, the emotional and the spontaneous characteristics of the movements rather than with any aesthetic orientation. It is an awakening through a pedagogical process of the possibilities for learning. It also works as a prophylaxis in preventing further disturbances in the child that essentially come from the society we are living in.

PMLD

Children with (PMLD) have a self-body that could develop along an atypical route but it is important to understand that this self-body is the root of their existence. Their movement may be highly restricted or erratic and deemed a behaviour problem. Many do not use formal communication rather make noises, gesture, use their faces which is their way of trying to be heard, there are different reasons for a child having a learning disability and there are different types: mild, moderate or severe. However, in all cases according to (Mencap, 2018) the child will be affected for their whole life.

ADHD

The clinical neuropsychologist Dr. Mario Martinez (2014, p. 195) calls "attention deficit disorder" an "abundance of curiosity" and while these conditions are thought to be genetic I tend to agree with him when he says that they are adaptations the child makes to the complex nature of living in these times. The child that is needing attention from his/her home for example can not only find refuge in a safe, playful space but can be heard, seen, met and understood in an environment of music, colour, activities, different props that allow him to speak intelligently away from the rigidity of the culture.

Through an emotion focused therapy programme for example these curious children are invited to play with total acceptance of whom, how and where they are in their difficult world. This empathic attunement to the child through movement and play enables the Therapist to discover his/her mode of learning, alleviate the anxiety and help make his/her experience of school a positive one where they are strong in their abilities to learn.

Dyspraxia

Is a condition where the normal process of physical actions is delayed in some way. Other ways to explain this is 'Developmental Co-ordination Disorder' or 'Clumsy Child Syndrome'. The child will have difficulty with his/her gross motor skills as well as his/her fine motor skills. This can be very frustrating for the child, their life very restricted which can often lead to isolation, bullying and strange behaviours. As the child grows older, they often-times develop more noticeable physical difficulties. Avoiding playground activities, walking up and down stairs; using scissors, writing and drawing; getting dressed or keeping still!
As one parent said to me many years ago:

> *"all it takes is going that extra step and reaching out with a hand, or an ear to listen or a smile, simple human things!"*

The sixth sense

The special Schools work with the learning-disabled child through a sensory educational programme that stimulates the five senses. However, they often forget the sixth one, the kinaesthetic one that is another channel for knowing and understanding life and one that is very much tops during the first infancy.

Learning disabilities are unseen and may run in families and recognising that the child or young person has a learning disability is very difficult because all the characteristics differ. However, taking action is the best thing you can do for them.

Receiving help in the early years is the best thing and really and improves their chances for succeeding. By identifying what it is that is causing your child's problems you are taking the first step toward help.

It can be scary for parents to come to terms with the fact that their child has a learning disability because of the hostility in the world however, you need not be afraid because with the right help you can realise that these children are just as intelligent as their peers it is simply that their brains are wired differently.

Some of the signs:

- Pronunciation problems
- Trouble learning numbers, words, colours
- Difficulty concentrating
- Difficulty interacting with peers
- Trouble following directions
- Trouble controlling pencil
- Difficulty with buttons etc.
- Confusing basic words
- Trouble learning about time
- Have trouble remembering facts
- Consistent reading and spelling errors
- Difficulty with letter sequencing
- Organising papers, bedroom desk
- Difficulty understanding discussions and expressing thought aloud
- Trouble with open ended questions on tests
- Trouble focusing on details
- Difficulty with a slow work pace
- Difficulty with spelling the same word differently

The learning-disabled child:

Movement says something about the child, his mood, his flexibility or rigidity and movement in relationship can enable him to change or at least to have a new experience or sensation. As an example, the child who has difficulties in completing schoolwork may not have a cognitive impairment at all. His / her learning difficulties may be a result of emotional stresses. The experience of joy and pleasure is fundamental throughout this approach and a good relationship with the therapist central to the process (Levy, 1988). In regards the needs of these children, these are understood as them needing a way to express their emotions and have the chance to address their communication problems (Karkou and Sanderson, 2000). The therapist working with learning disabled child places prime importance on the development of the body image. Having a good background in dance, they use praise and touch. Praise in the context of person-centred therapy where the empowerment of the individual is paramount through the core conditions (Rogers, 1980) of unconditional positive regard, congruence and empathy. That is, avoiding disempowering attitudes in the relationship.

Stress and the parent

Here are some findings gathered from my research study a few years ago which highlight the need for helping parents in concrete ways.

Stress is a big factor in their lives and according to (Walton, 1993) they just have the experience of being unable to cope. They worry they are not doing enough for their child according to (Smith, 2002),often the child's disability puzzles them because they do not know how much of it is due to the nature of the condition and how much it is the child being in opposition to them. It seems that the most difficult part for parents in raising a child with autism is the social implications of their child's behaviour. That is their lack of responsiveness socially and how it affects them socially too (Ludlow, A. et al., 2011).

In 'Disability & society refocusing on the parent': (Case, 2000) urges professionals to teach them their skills, in order that they might become more competent and skilled themselves. Saying, in addition, those parents provide valuable insights into their child's social situation.

Moreover, in a study conducted in 2010 on 'The Experiences of Parents with Adolescents Identified as Having a Specific Learning Disability' (Seals, 2010), listening to the parents was seen as paramount. Their perspective is now seen as an essential element in the journey to understanding their own needs and experiences as well as their child's (Read, 2000).

A study made in Australia acknowledges that the perspectives of the child with learning disabilities are essential too (Garth and Aroni, 2003). However, we cannot ask a child with (PMLD) directly but we can do the next best thing and ask those who know them well (Sheehy and Nind, 2005).

Parents of children with learning disabilities live with prejudices and discriminations. This preoccupation in our society with levels of disability seems Cartesian as some disabled children are open to investigation, i.e. those with mild learning difficulties and others are left in the arena of irreversible, individualised biology, with severe learning disabilities as (Goodley, 2001) points out.

In conclusion, the stress of the parents seems huge. They worry about the child's lack of ability to socialise and have high levels of anxiety, perhaps feeling guilty because they wonder and blame themselves for their child's difficulties and behaviours. The studies also show that parents need to be listened to and suggest professionals teach them their skills.
So, having ideas to work with and skill building sessions is a simple doable way to help you as a parent / carer.

Time of the diagnosis

As I mentioned briefly many parents experience deep grief when they realise that they have a child with additional needs. Some studies of the effects on the attachment system of an early diagnosis of a learning disability point to the fact that the attachment will probably be insecure (Esterhuyzen & Hollins, 1977) here there is an insecure attachment between the mother and the child which is a result of the learning disability, the disability can be experienced as a trauma at the time of the diagnosis and also at the time when the child him/herself becomes cognitively aware of it.

The three internalised styles of insecure attachment are:

- Avoidant – where the client moves away from hostile parents and believes they are better off alone; the baby feels so uncomfortable with others who are not nourishing.
- Ambivalent – where the child gets inconsistent love and has had caregivers who are unpredictable. The baby feels a lack of sense of self and tries to get it from another
- Disorganized – is both of the above and with a lack of sense of safety and security from deep in their physiology

What can you do as caretaker of the child / adult to restore and embody secure attachment skills?
With a child who has Avoidant attachment you need to let them know you understand that things are better on their own but explore what it will be like to allow others to share with you. For example, Shall we do this together? Here, the key is to work with the "importance of including other"

- With a child who has ambivalent attachment you would help them come back to a sense of self (the key). Help them refer to themselves. "Close your eyes and go into to yourself, what do you think?"
- With disorganised you need to focus on safety and regulating the central nervous system to feel a sense of physiological safety inside. Who/what provides that sense of safety for them and where in the body is this. The key is creating body-felt sense of safety and relaxation.

When we experience secure attachment we are able to live in deeper compassion and intimacy. We don't suffer post-traumatic stress disorders; we recover from stress easier and experience brain integration.
Tips to help you:

1. Connect, connect, connect
2. Make the child client the centre of the universe
3. Embody safety
4. Separate, connect. Separate, connect
5. Remember you don't need a special talent to love and hold in safety

Mirror Neurons

As a Movement Psychotherapist myself I know that techniques such as mirroring work with individuals with learning disabilities because they reach them through activating the Mirror Neuron System and revitalising the body sensations. Establishing that sense of trust in themselves and in the other. Helping with social skills and providing an outlet for discharge of tension, frustrations and hostilities.
Neuroscience shows us how emotion focused movement embraces the most important aspects of the child because it is not only through mirroring and witnessing movement that identical sets of neurons can be activated but by being in the action or the expression of the feeling, behaviour. The Mirror Neuron System, when sparked, enables the child/adult grow and learn.
The Mirroring Technique is as old as time as it is the way we make friends and know those closest to us. It is often an unconscious behaviour that makes your relationships stronger and tells the other that you can be trusted. There is a mirror neuron system in the brain that is to do with emotional empathy and it is said that empathy is developed when these neurons fire with another. Many people believe that those with autism have a mirror neurons system that misfires and this is why difficulties with empathy, social skills; understanding others' motives etc. arise. However, this has not been proven completely to be the case.
Mirror Neuron System is activated through engagement with others either through play, pedagogy and socialising and most children/adults like to learn with others, be part of others rather than being alone. The technique of mirroring an individual's movement can be applied to establish trust and build the therapeutic relationship, which is nurtured sensitively through the therapists' ability to mirror, echo, sustain, follow and enlarge the child's movement range and expressions.

Dance Movement Psychotherapists are trained to be sensitive to movement language as it relates to the psychological, motor and cognitive development.

Containing and Safety

Donald Winnicott, a British Paediatrician and Psychoanalyst, speaks about the holding environment, the safe space which goes all the way back to what happens between mother and baby hence, the importance of this.

The potential space or transitional space depends on experiences that lead to trust, a "sacred place" from where the baby experiences creative living. So, having compassion, empathy and being consistent and trustworthy will ensure that you are providing the necessary safe place.

As learning-disabled children frequently engage in idiosyncratic patterns of moving (Levy, 1988) meeting them in their movement patterns through dance and rhythm is a way to build the relationship.

Playing is a creative expression that bridges the inner and the outer worlds.

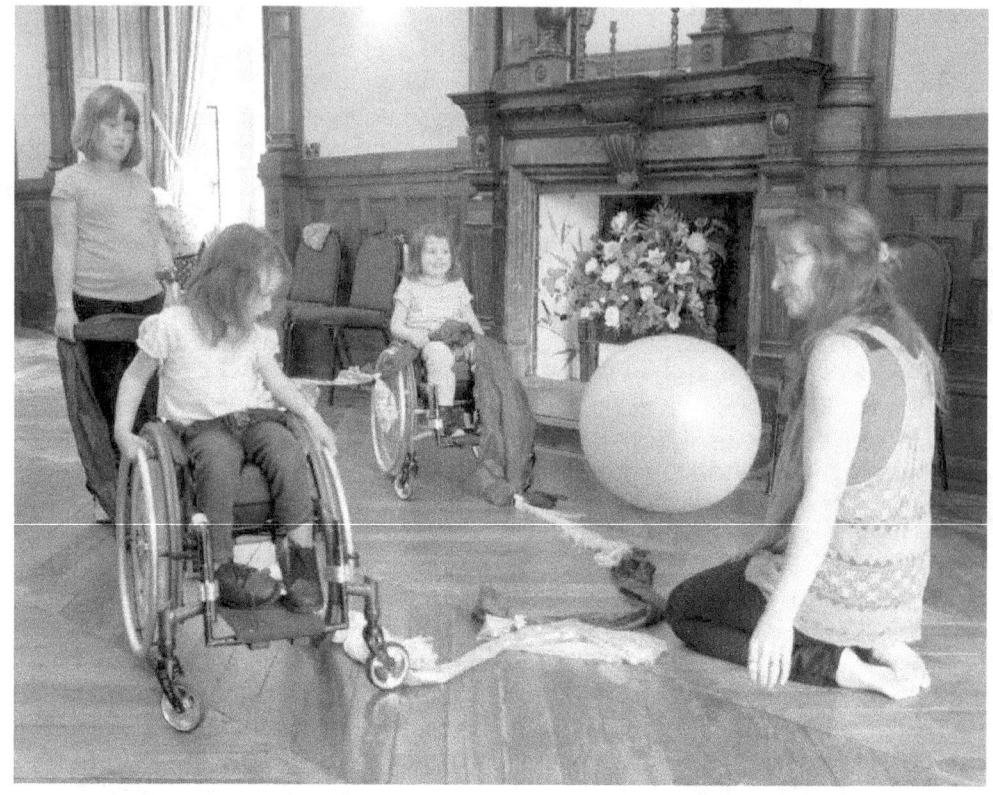

"The goal of this 'play therapy' experience is to afford an opportunity for formless experience and for creating impulses, motor and sensory, which are the stuff of playing and on the basis of playing is built the whole of man's existence"

Winnicott, 1971, p.75)

Being a real person for the individual with learning disabilities is like the role of the therapist. So, as the carer you could begin to see yourself a little as a therapist and be that real person. This is one of the invitations of this book.

When a mother and baby attune to each other's needs then empathy develops and then the baby understands that they are wanted, seen enough and have that necessary foundation from which to grow. Without this catastrophic consequences are the result.

"As with looking, so with holding. Not just the physical holding of the baby by the mother but the entire psychophysiological system of protection, support, caring and containing that envelops the child, without which it would not survive

(Holmes, 1993)

It is also necessary to imagine yourself as the mother with the responsibility of providing for your children good quality experiences where you are allowing exploration and expression as oppose to rigid rules and expectations.
If you are not a mother this does not matter! Staying present with an open heart allows the safety base to be built. Safety is a fundamental key to our clients / patients' journey towards what ultimately must be more of a joyful connection with life.

Neuroscience, Dance and Autism - Neuroscience Research and Dance Movement Psychotherapy

Neuroscience is the study of the nervous system – including the brain, the spinal cord, and networks of sensory nerve cells, or neurons, throughout the body. Humans contain roughly 100 billion neurons, the functional units of the nervous system (Neuroscience, 2012).

Antonio Damasio is a neuroscientist who recognises that the mind is not a sophisticated tool separate from the rest of the body. He suggests that what the mind experiences as an emotion is really a group of somatic cues that he calls 'somatic markers' which include blood flow, hormone levels, digestive activity, neurotransmitters and other areas of cellular metabolism (Damasio, 1994: 165). One of the characteristics of children on the autistic spectrum is actively avoiding relationships thus, withdrawing into their own world. Therapeutic interventions engaging relational experience and expressive communication are consistent with the work of movement psychotherapy (Homann, 2010: 91).

A fundamental concept of neuroscience is that the mirror matching mechanism of the brain is activated when relating to stimuli outside of the self, when in relationship with another. This specialized group of brain cells is located in the parts of the brain that respond to sensorimotor stimuli, to stimulation of the senses (Berrol, 2006: 307). To understand an illness that concurrently involves interruptions of gait, eye contact, and language as well the ability for abstract reasoning, one must be attentive to the interrelationship of systems that comprise the central nervous system (CNS) as many levels of neural processing are involved
(Cozolino, 2006: 284)

When the therapist is witnessing a client in movement, the mirror matching networks within the (CNS) are generating interneuronal connectivity between them both (Berrol, 2006: 308).

The vagus nerve controls the parasympathetic nervous system that is paramount in resting. Functioning of this nerve is influenced in early development through the quality of touch experienced from caregivers (Hart, 2008).
However, an autistic brain functions differently from one that is perfectly healthy. The cells in the limbic circuits of the brain are not as developed as in a healthy brain. Panskepp suggests that autistic aloofness may be the product of the basic

emotional systems of the brain, which are moulded during early development, not receiving the care, love and nurture needed for healthy development (Panksepp, 2001: 13).

The somatic attunement of the movement therapist through embodied movement activates the mirror neuron system, and through neuronal, hormonal and chemical cascades connecting the limbic, autonomous nervous system and right hemisphere's orbitofrontal cortex, facilitates experiences of being with another. Because this process activates early relational attachments, it is fundamental in psychotherapeutic work (Homann, 2010: 90).

"The period from 7 to 15 months is considered optimal for receiving particular affective stimuli in the portions of the brain undergoing rapid development. It is a time when axonal myelination, dendritic proliferation and connectivity are facilitating the maturation of the limbic and cortical association areas, a time when attachment patterns are forming." (Berrol, 2006: 310)

Mirroring the baby, the mother stimulates the neurological pathways of the brain building empathy, the ability to understand and experience the emotional world of other. Conceived of as a mental state it is dependent on right hemispheric resources (Decety and Chaminade, 2003).
As body awareness through rhythmic activities and relaxing emphasising one body part at a time were some of the interventions employed with the children affective self-regulation was being encouraged.

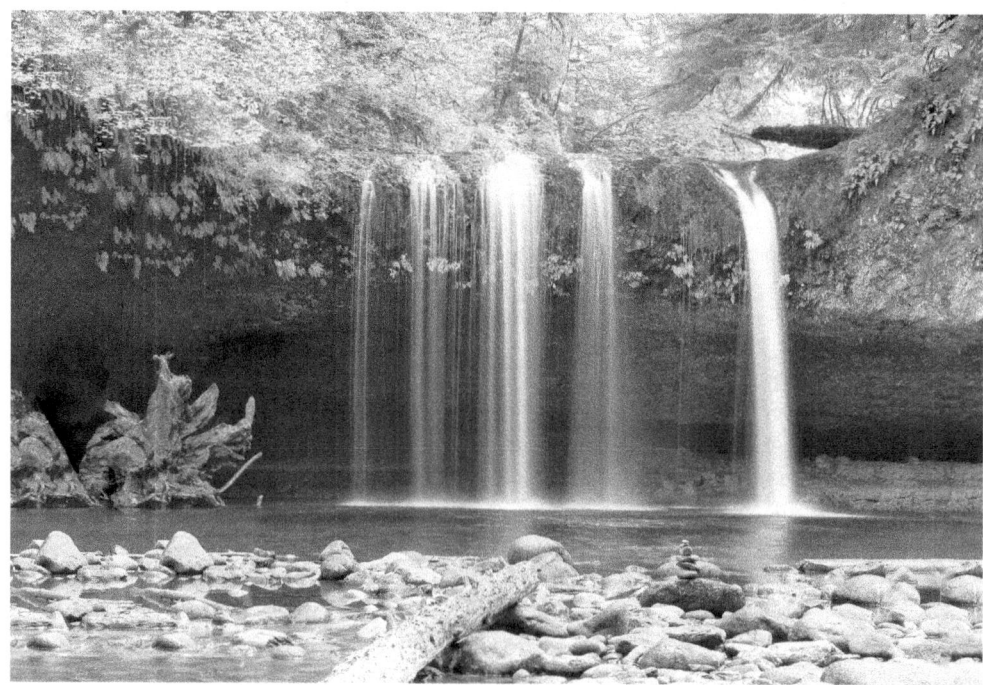

Waterfall - by Pixabay - Free-Photos

PART TWO

'Connecting with your body and spirit is an essential part of self-care'

This second chapter of the book offers exercises to do at home, meditations for one to come home and reconnect into your own body and spirit in just minutes as well as exercises that you can do with your child / friend when you are together. Love and creativity are two forces in everybody's life that if we allow them to move through us show us our true nature and identity and the identity that we have been educated into through the culture dissolves.

Love flow

The first exercise is a ` Love flow' Self-healing meditation to be done when you have 10 minutes to be alone in a place where you will not be disturbed. I suggest you read it through a few times and then go through it. You could record it and

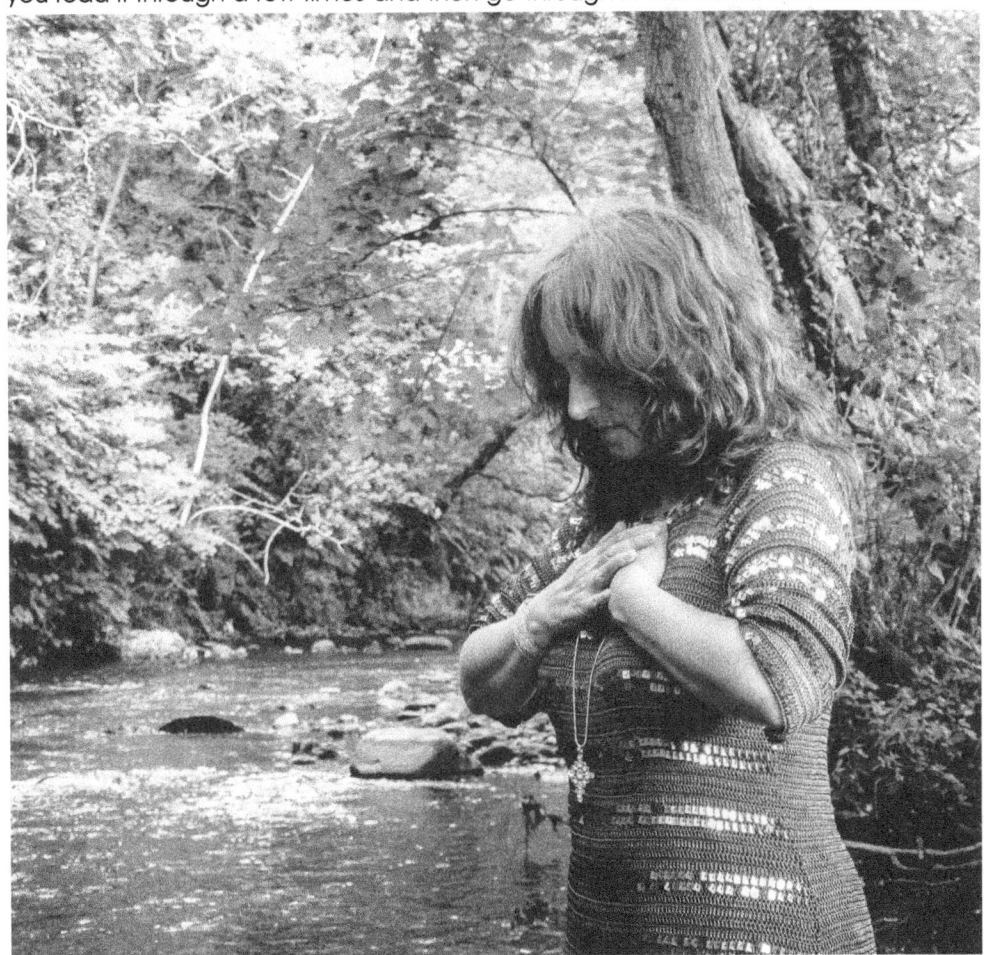

then listen to your own voice guiding you through! Play some gentle music in the background and get yourself a warm drink and settle in.

We are going to connect with the energetics of your body system and using visualization allow yourself to trust the sensations and images that may arise. The energy that runs through your body is very subtle and has a very gentle voice. It can be pictured as a light and runs through different channels and centres and points within your body. Many of you will know these centres as chakras, meridians or other energetic systems within the body for example. Through learning to use your fine energy you are focusing as well on the energy of your heart and thus helping compassion to grow. If you do this you are better able to attune to the energy of your child / friend.

The breathing is a big guide here and I urge you to breathe in for four, hold for four, exhale for four and repeat this until you begin to feel anxiety free and more yourself before you begin.

- Sitting in a comfortable chair or lying down quiet yourself; unwind by taking a few deep breaths until you are feeling centred. Gently place your hand over your heart in the mid-chest. Tap a few times on your heart centre as if you are inviting it to connect with you. See your heart in your mind's eye beating as you breathe and slow down. Breathe into the bottom of the heart, to the top and all sides.

- Focus on; bring to mind someone or something that makes you feel the energy of love, a person, an animal or a memory from the past. Relax into this and allow the energy of your heart to flood you.

- Next, feel into your physical sensations body and explore what or how are you feeling right now? Do you feel physical pain or discomfort? Are your muscles tight?

  Is their tightness in your throat, your heart or your chest?
  Is there holding in your shoulders, are they scrunched up towards your ears?
  How is your belly?
  What are the muscles feeling like in your legs?
  Is your jaw clenched tight?
  Your eyes?
  Do you feel physical pain in your spine?
  How is the bottom of your spine in your pelvis?

Notice any images that arise and taking your time scan through your entire body

- Ask yourself where you need loving attention.

- Once you have done a body and emotional scan send the energy of your heart to those places in your body that are in need of love. Breathe in through your heart and as you breathe out do so to the places that needs your gentle heart energy. See this as a colour if this feels right.

- Next send this heart energy out to others. Bring to mind someone who needs kindness, understanding whatever they need and send this energy out in the form of a colour, perhaps green or pink or whatever feels right to you. Do this a few times and enjoy it.

- You don't need to force this, you just need to let it flow, let love flow! See the people you are reaching out to touch with this loving energy receiving this and then come back to yourself

- Wiggle your fingers and toes, open your eyes and thank your heart for that journey.

Affection

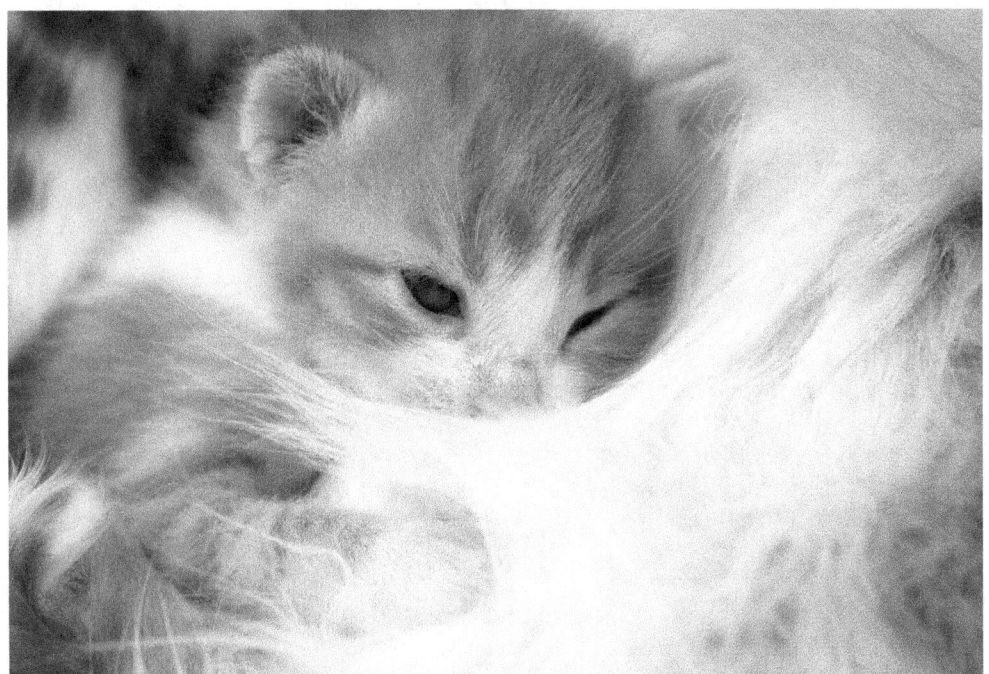

Kitten - Pixabay by Antonio Doumas

What we are interested in is giving and receiving tenderness on a daily basis and keeping this flow of energy open. This is what connects us all, not competition, or doctorates; not clever words or money but, Love. You all understand this and know this to be true in your heart and souls. You were born without hatred in your heart but this is what gets taught to us in one way or another.

"No one is born hating another person because of the colour of his skin, or his background, or his religion. People must learn to hate, and if they can learn to hate, they can be taught to love, for love comes more naturally to the human heart than its opposite"

(Nelson Mandela, 1994)

Affection or empathy, love is in one way or another connected to the world of feelings; of sensations, body intuitions. It is through this flow that we build deep affinities with others and find a pathway that comes from our hearts. The biology of love is related with the instinct of intra-species solidarity, altruism and bonding rituals.

We live in a world where love, affection, sweetness and solidarity have become alien. How did this happen? The way to change this is to change ourselves.

Heartmath researchers have found that when people focus their attention on the heart and activate a core heart feeling, such a love, and appreciation; gratitude, compassion and caring that these emotions immediately shift their heartbeat rhythms into more coherent patterns, thus we are more able to act from the heart.

The genius of our species is not intelligence, it is affection, sweetness and empathy; that is orientated towards tolerance, compassion, friendship and love which is what we need urgently flowing through our bodies and families and communities and planet

Mirroring

The second exercise is Mirror in Movement game to do with your child / friend at home or wherever you may be with space enough to move around in. So, for this exercise you will need a big enough space, cleared from clutter and pleasant to spend time in. You will need a good music system that is clear and of good quality. The aim of this exercise is to work with colour in play and movement. You will need approx. 20 to 30 minutes.

- As the leader you are going to play a nice rhythmic piece of music and moving around the space and tapping different body parts, 'let's say hello to our shoulders', then let's say hello to our legs and moving around the body.

- After moving through the body you then call out one body part to focus on and put a word to that body part. Repeat this several times.

- Now choosing another piece of music you are going to ask your child / friend to choose one part and move to the music with this. As they begin to move around you are going to mirror their dance and guess what it might be saying.

- How to do this?

- Take a little distance

- Gently follow the smallest movement

- After a time introduce a sound to their movement or respond to the energy of their dance with a movement that is similar in feel.

- Have fun!

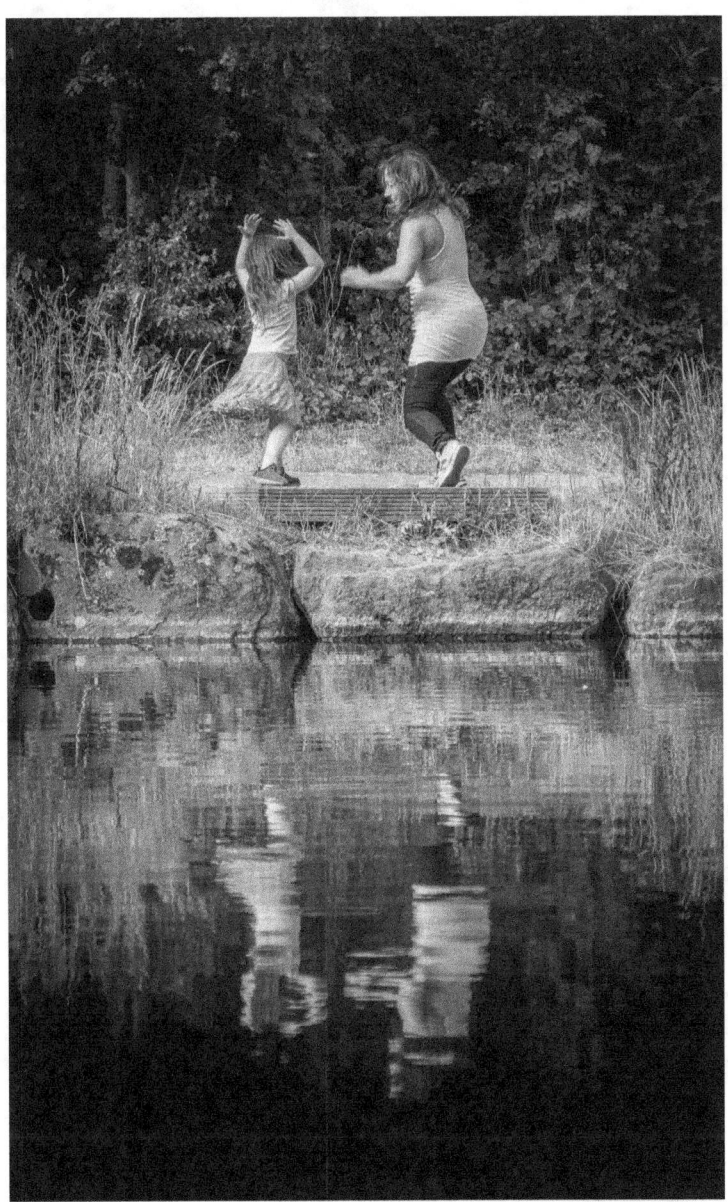

Presence

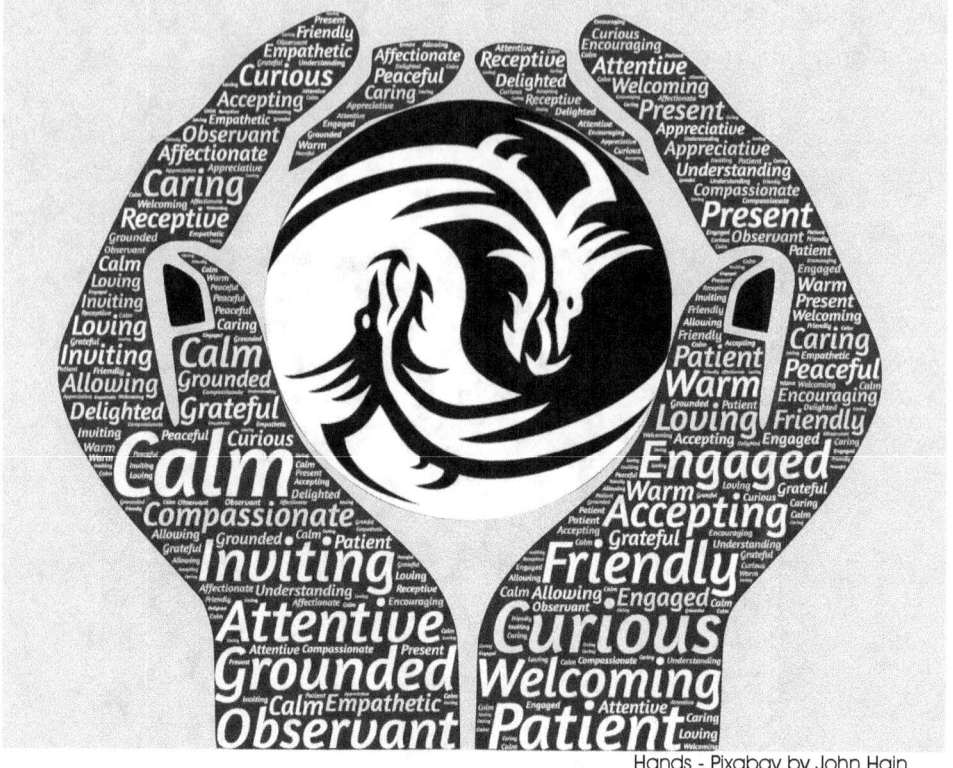

Hands - Pixabay by John Hain

Love has many arms. For example really listening to and being present with our child / friend is how we can love them. We have a tendency in our culture to believe that if someone is talking to us and sharing themselves that we need to come up with a solution for them because we think that it will make them feel better and we feel better because we think we have helped someone. But, we have not helped them; we have just stroked our own ego and disregarded what they have said really.

Often-times in organisations or schools, day centres the child / friend with special needs can get lost in the hub bub of the dramas presented by those who are caring for them. Even in one to one situations or sessions, very often I have witnessed kind people engaging with these individuals through art, or movement, or some creative activity; but their "quality of presence" is not there. It is very subtle but it is not there!

If you are present, you are more able to know what your child / friend needs/feels and is communicating in their way.

"It is the quality of presence that grants presence"

Honesty

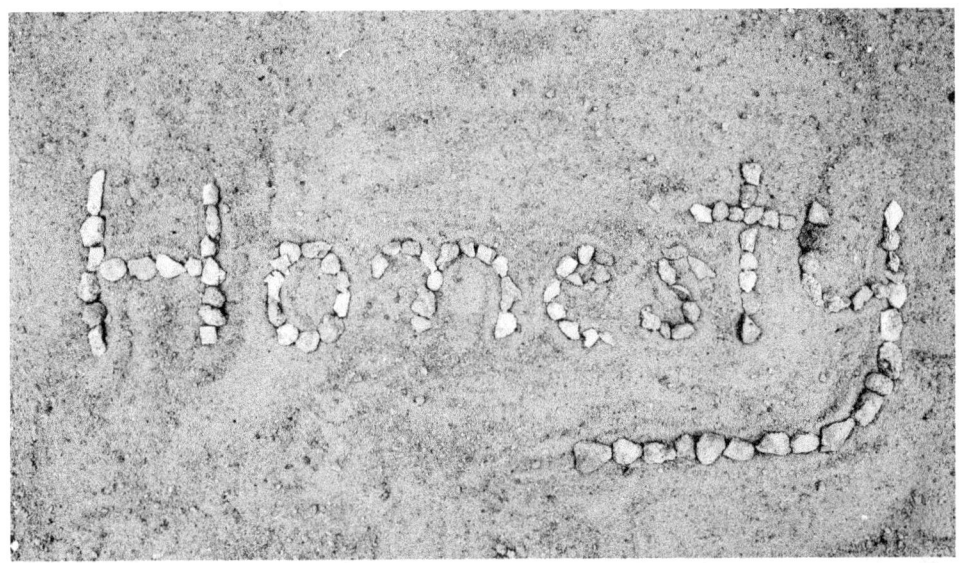

Honesty - Pixabay by Muhammad Haseeb Muhammad Suleman

The third exercise is exploring what self-care means to you through an 'Ask your body Meditation'. Part of a self-care practice is having clear boundaries and being honest with yourself and others. Honouring your own needs and not giving away your time and energy to anyone and everyone because sooner or later you will suffer as a result through illness or relationship breakdowns or loss of creativity. Be honest with yourself, in your feeling emotional system. Asking yourself things like "why do I feel angry here"; or "what is my body telling me"; or "what do I need"?

- Find a comfortable place to sit or lie down. Inhale to the count of four, hold for the count of four, exhale for the count of four, hold for the count of four and REPEAT three or four times. This should really slow you down and bring to centredness.

- Next, continuing with slow and steady breathing ask yourself, how am I feeling, what am I feeling, what is my body trying to tell me?

- Accepting what arises is the first thing you must pay attention to; recognising that this is being honest towards yourself.

- Inwardly and in a relaxed state continue with this enquiry, breathing in and out. If you start to feel anxious because you cannot connect into a feeling or sensation inside it is very important not to be harsh on yourself but to just accept that this is how it is for you in this moment.

- Don't force, just invite.

This exercise can last for 10 mins.

- Grab a pen and paper and write from the felt sense in your body i.e. images, memories, sensations etc.

- You don't need to be concerned with grammar or spelling at all!

- Journaling is a good way to get your thoughts and emotions out without having to verbalise them. It is a great way to bring your inner world outside and offers a way of clear perspective and too spiritual insight.

- Set the timer for ten minutes and write away!

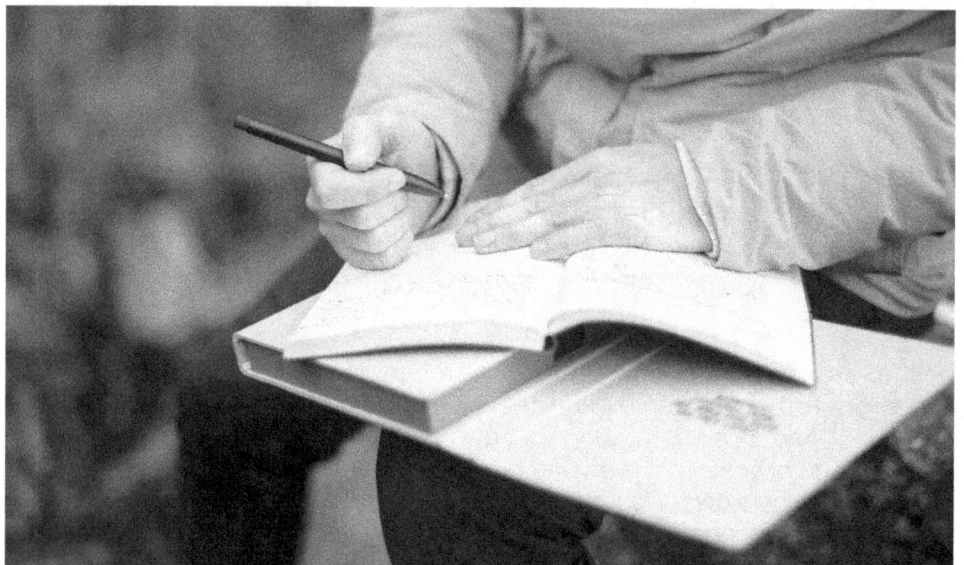

Adult - Pixabay by Pexels

"Many writers, poets, and certainly journal writers have always intuitively known that writing can heal"
(Susan Borkin, 2014, p.3)

- Are you going to begin a self-care practice....10 mins per day?

The Language of Touch

From the heartbeat of our mother that we hear when in the womb we begin receiving tactile signals. So it is of no wonder then that touch plays such a critical part in the parent-child relationship right from the beginning: "It's an essential channel of communication with caregivers for a child," says San Diego State University School of Communication emeritus professor Peter Andersen.
A mothers touch enhances the attachment and bonding with her and her child and can say: "you are safe, I'm here". It can generate positive or negative emotions depending on the context because a squeeze can signal a warning to not touch a certain object. A mothers touch can help mitigate the pain of having a blood test and touch in form of massage has so many benefits such as improving sleep, helping digestion; lowering the blood pressure, promoting muscle relaxation; improve circulation, reduce stress; strengthen the body's immune system and restore your posture.
The culture plays a role and also the home and social environment too. If you are from a religious family perhaps you were taught that touch is sinful and inappropriate because this is what some of the religions teach. Spend time in a different culture or with friends who are touchy-feely and your attitude might change.

By the time we're adults, we realise that touch connects us. In research done back in 1976, clerks at a university library returned library cards to students either with or without briefly touching the student's hand. Student interviews revealed that those who'd been touched evaluated the clerk and the library more favourably. The effect held even when students hadn't noticed the touch.

The Effects of Contact and touch at Organic and Existential level

The neurophysiological effects of touch studied by Rene Spitz in hospitalised children marked a revolution in paediatrics. New research showed that touch activate the cardio-respiratory system, dissolve chronic defence motor tensions and reinforce the immune system. According to Wilhelm Reich(1993), an Austrian Doctor touch diminishes sexual repression and tendencies to authoritarianism. It increases the self-esteem and strengthens the identity.

Spitz discovered that children who had been institutionalised particularity in the first months of their lives lacking maternal affection, experienced irreversible damage in the motor and affective aspects, in the language and intellectual developmental Germaine Greer in her work "The Neurosis of Abandonment" states that affective de-valorisation is only observed in people who lacked love and understanding during their early infancy

E. Kaila: "Die reaktion des Sauglings auf das menschliche Gesicht" demonstrated that when the child does not smile at three months in front of a human face or that he reacts negatively and with screams, maternal care has been defective or non existent. (experiences confirmed by Spitz)

Kunz pointed out that if the affective touch is a confirmation needed by the other, the smile is the confirmation of the 'being seen in the encounter and the possibility of getting on well, syntonic salvation.

Rof Carballo proposes that the smile is the first psychosocial reflection and that its neurological meaning is that neurological maturation of the cortical-diencephalic paths has normally occurred. If the child has not smiled at three months old he/she is seriously ill.

Studies on "Transitional Object" realised by Freud, Winnicott, Lapierre and Piaget demonstrated that children creatively try out their 'separation and encounter' with objects that have an affective meaning for them and it is in this way that they develop and reinforce their identity.

Arnold Gessell described the evolution of the personal-social behaviour of children and its sexual and affective manifestations from birth to teenage. It is one of the most objective studies on the development of natural impulses to contact and affective communication

Frederick Le-boyer "For a Birth without Violence" stresses the importance of contact on the baby's body and says that through contact with the hands the child registers everything: nervousness or calm, awkwardness or security, tenderness or violence. He / she knows if the hands love him, or if they are distracted or worse if they are rejecting him
If faced with uncaring and hostile hands, he/she isolates himself, withdraws from the world and closes up. So, before following the waves that run through his little body it is enough to rest ones hands without any movement at all onto the child.
The hands must not be distracted hands, absent or inert. But present, attentive and alive following the subtle movements of the child. Light and soft hands, not authoritarian ones rather hands that do not ask for anything, they are simply present.
Hands full of tenderness and silence

Touch and Movement

The language of movement is one of the most primitive forms of expression and perception for infants, it is the first mode of understanding as the vestibular nerves that are responsible for the registering of movement are the first ones to develop in utero. Movement therefore has an important role in "establishing the baseline" for other perceptual processes (Cohen, 1987)

According to the Father of Modern Dance Rudolf Laban the realm of physical sensation and intention is related to the element of weight. The quality of the first relationship with the mother's body will establish a foundation for that infant for how she/he will experience his/her own body through her lifetime. The skin, the body's largest and most vital sensory organ is the pathway or channel if you like of earliest communication. The skin to skin contact with the mother, this sense of touch gives rise to the experience of the ego (Anzieu, 1989).

"If somebody feels invaded by touch we need to listen to their feelings of invasion and give them a space to express and release their feelings, make their own boundaries so that they firstly develop a sense of safety within their own body" (Jill Hayes, 2013)

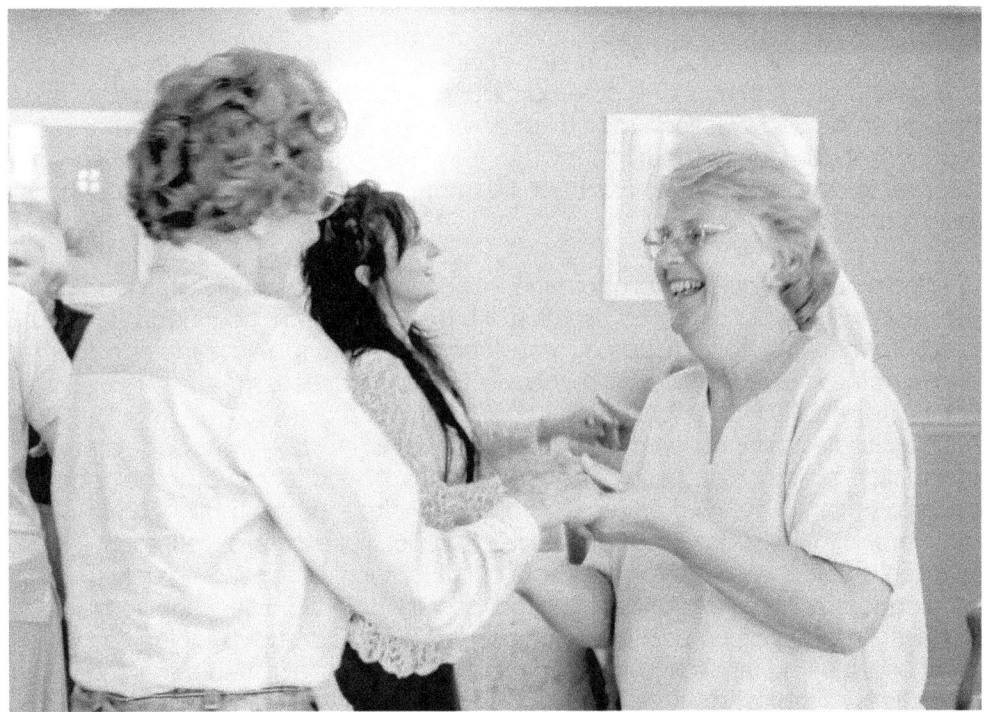

In person-centred practice empathy is a core condition understood to be the quality of being able to walk in someone's shoes knowing that I am into him/her. It is the ability to let the others life resonate inside my own. In Movement psychotherapy mirroring is part of the process and it is vital that they arise as an authentic emphatic response. Mirroring is not simply copying another persons movement but a very subtle process of being involved in the others movement. A movement of soul to soul communication.

The (DMP) therapist working with learning disabled child places prime importance on the development of the body image. Having a good background in dance, they use praise and touch. Praise in the context of person-centred therapy where the empowerment of the individual is paramount through the core conditions (Rogers, 1980) of unconditional positive regard, congruence and empathy. That is, avoiding disempowering attitudes in the relationship.

We learn about the world through our bodies

It is through our bodies that we know the world. It is through our bodies that we know other people and I believe this is the same for every human and animal too! We do not think first and then know the world, rather we learn about it through movement. The baby starts to move and stretch in responses to pleasure or pain. we don't have to think if we are hungry or not, or think if we like someone or not; or if we are tired or need comfort, protection, friendship etc.

When there is a full embodied connection that is helped to grow, that is watered and given warmth through the core conditions that Carl Rogers taught us and through embodied presence (as it is not enough just to have empathy you need a body that can contain your clients) then they have a beautiful opportunity to discover and recover (if there has been trauma) themselves and others through their feeling body system.

"Our instinctual feeling-programs are the foundation for what allows us to plan and move ahead with purpose and direction. It is the fabric of what connects us to one another. When this critical map becomes disordered and maladaptive with trauma or protracted stress, as a consequence, we simply become lost"
Peter A. Levine, PhD (IN AN Unspoken Voice)
A full embodied connection means that the therapist has her whole body attuned to the client's feelings and emotional experiences. It is the tendency to balance and integrating of the different aspects of the self, the sensory,emotional and the mental (Katya Bloom, The Embodied Self, 2006). For example, your client may feel so alive when playing with balls but they stop this because it is silly, it is not academic; it is not reaching educational or therapeutic assessment levels. However, what it is doing as a physiological and biological level is lightening the heart and showing the way towards connection, containment, understanding and love because that is how it is being held. And this is something that is registered in the body.

The culture, society is very mind orientated towards thinking about and intellectualising everything, we can see this in our schools, churches and clubs. The heart has been taken out of everything! We all learn to navigate the culture and society we are born into and for those with learning disabilities' and trauma of some kind navigating these stormy seas must be terrifying. It's terrifying for the healthiest of us so imagine what it is like if you have additional needs.

As an example someone with disabilities may feel very shy precisely because of their disability. A speech and language therapist may say that this person does not like to move their body to music, they are shy and therefore it is not good for them. But, deep inside the person is an ancestral, primitive need to dance and be seen, it is what makes their heart jump with joy! But nobody knows this, they have never told anyone, they have learnt to hide because of their disability and on top of this are in a culture that is working from the mindset of do, go get more, be the best, reach higher, work harder and not from the heart, of acceptance, joy, togetherness, celebration and union. So, the heart says yes to playing and dancing and the school and therapist say no its okay you don't need to if you are shy rather than being able to see what it is really that their heart wants to do and allowing this pathway to life to open up.

Often-times it is only in experiencing this form of Movement therapy that one realises and understands through their body that indeed they like it, either in a playful moment, a spontaneous movement; a flowing movement or a silent still position or in the sharing. When the heart is given the space to jump with joy then this is a moment that has the potential for that person to feel life, to know life, their basic human right.

Sign language too is another brilliant language but it is not the language of the heart. The non-verbal world is the realm that we are working into through these movement psychotherapy sessions and it is here in the body that the pre-verbal material can be accessed. So for me it is a way of working with the whole of the person that reaches the body and the soul to access what came here to be expressed, the unique gifts inside each person.

Having fun through drama and stories is good for confidence building and bringing people together but what really matters is that the voice of the heart is understood, heard and nurtured in a way where they realise creativity in all the little things in their life, not just in the production of a story or play or in the making of masks for example. But, where they feel solidarity, friendship and the need for care; to realise that the vital energy of the person is their immune system functioning, realise that the spirituality is very important and is given a pathway through which to journey with this.

Body Movement

The deeper level of tuning into someone happens through subtle bodily sensations and postures through speed alignment and shaping of the body. It happens through sensing muscle tone, voice tone, intensities and timings.

Exercise number four is to help you tune into your child / friend through movement. You will need space enough to move around in and Music to guide you.

- The activity consists of sitting cross legged opposite each other as close as possible.

- Holding hands and breathing together, from time to time and when it feels right to look into each other's eyes from the gentle energy of your heart.

- As the leader you will step away and begin a movement sequence / patterning / dynamic / gesture / sound that shows your child / friend how you are feeling today. You will repeat this three times and then sit back opposite your partner holding hands and breathing together.

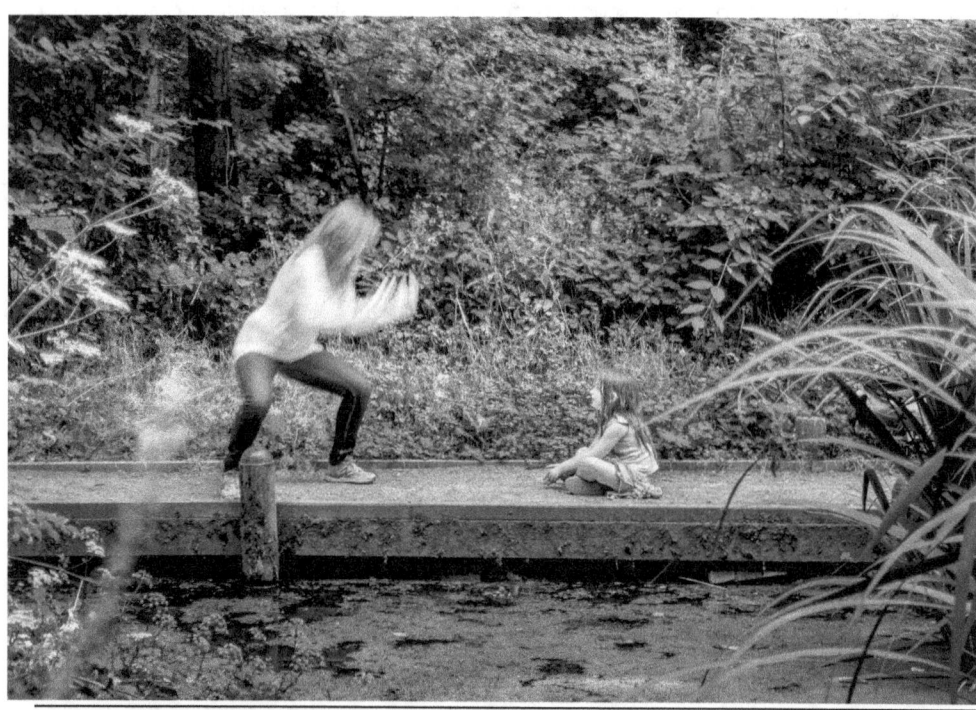

Karen Woodley - Movement Psychotherapy – RDMP

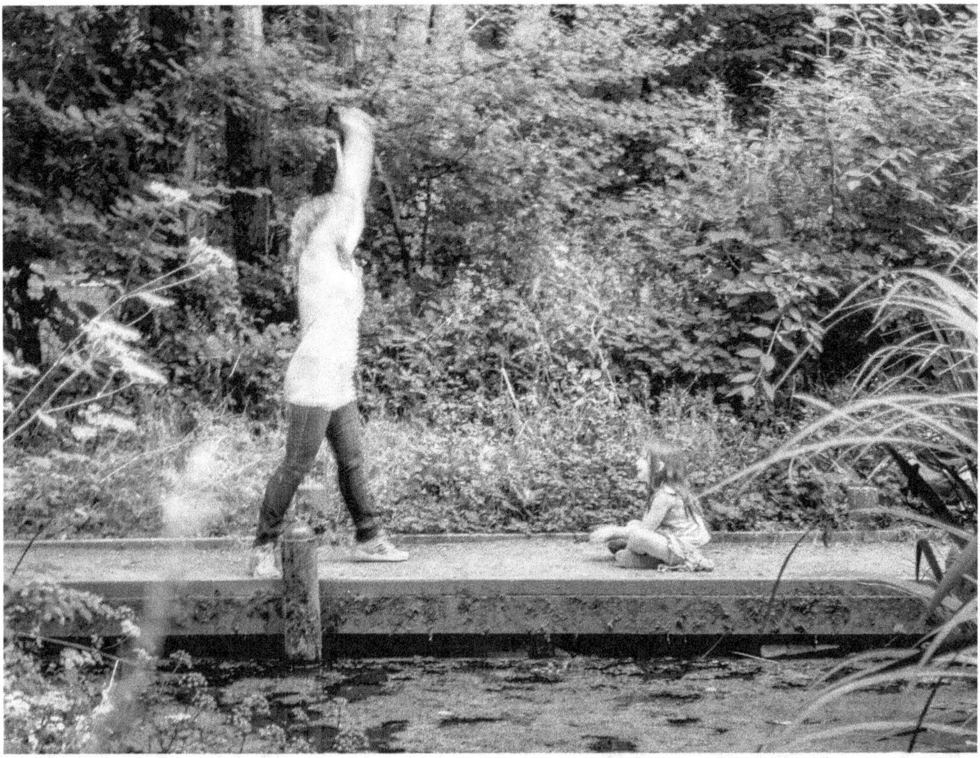

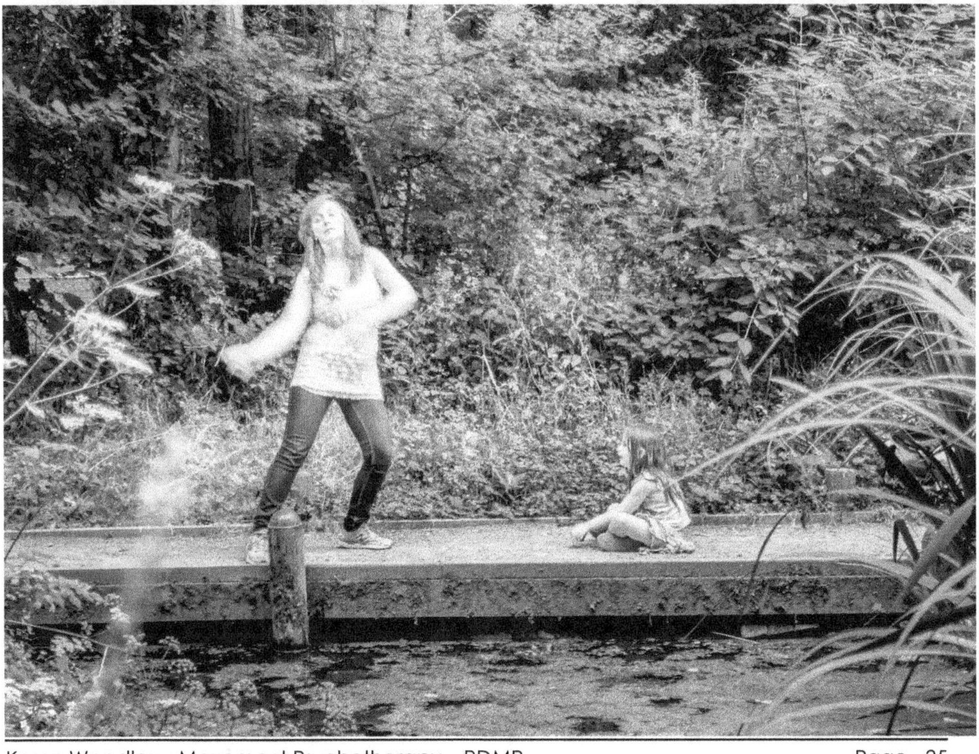

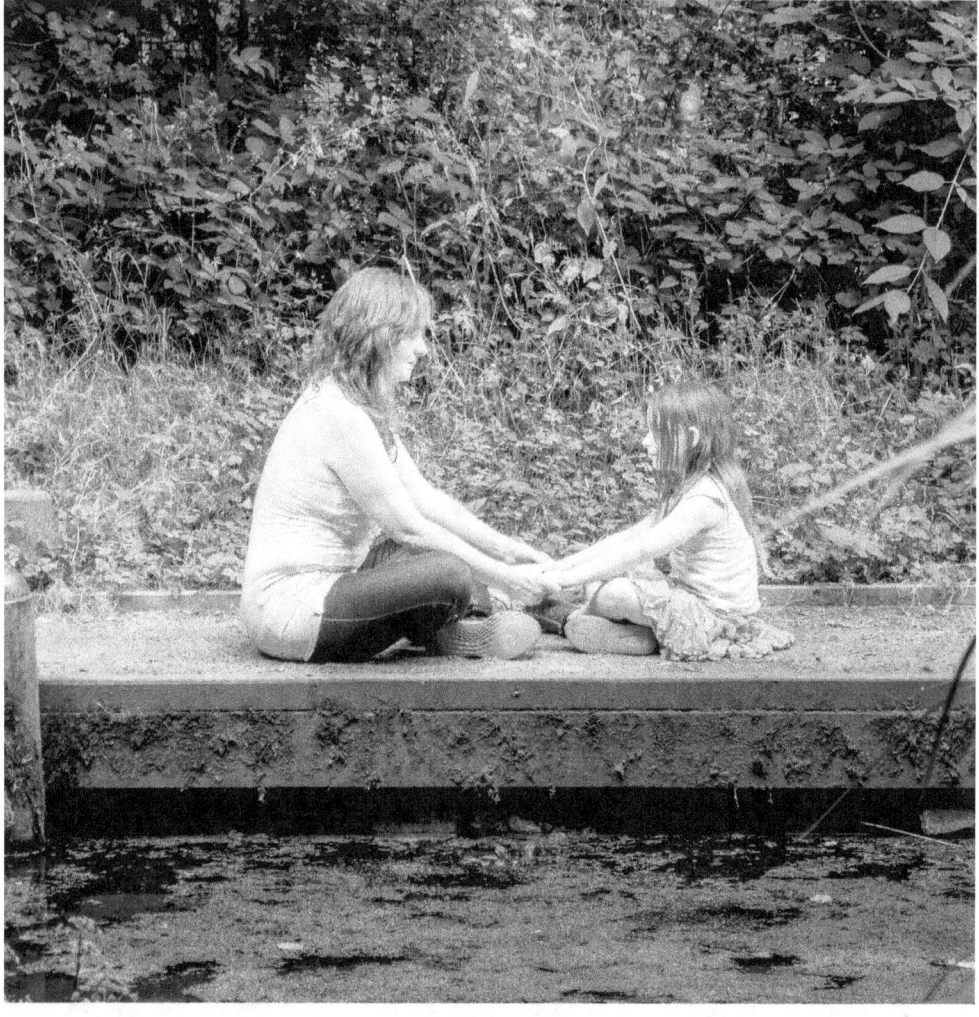

- Next it is your partners turn to express him/herself through their non-verbal movement patterning and shaping in the space. Again, repeating this three times and settling back down together.

- As the leader you will be noticing inner sensation and intuitions as they arise being mindful of images and feelings.

- What was that like for you? Perhaps share this experience together and set a time to go over this exercise again next week.

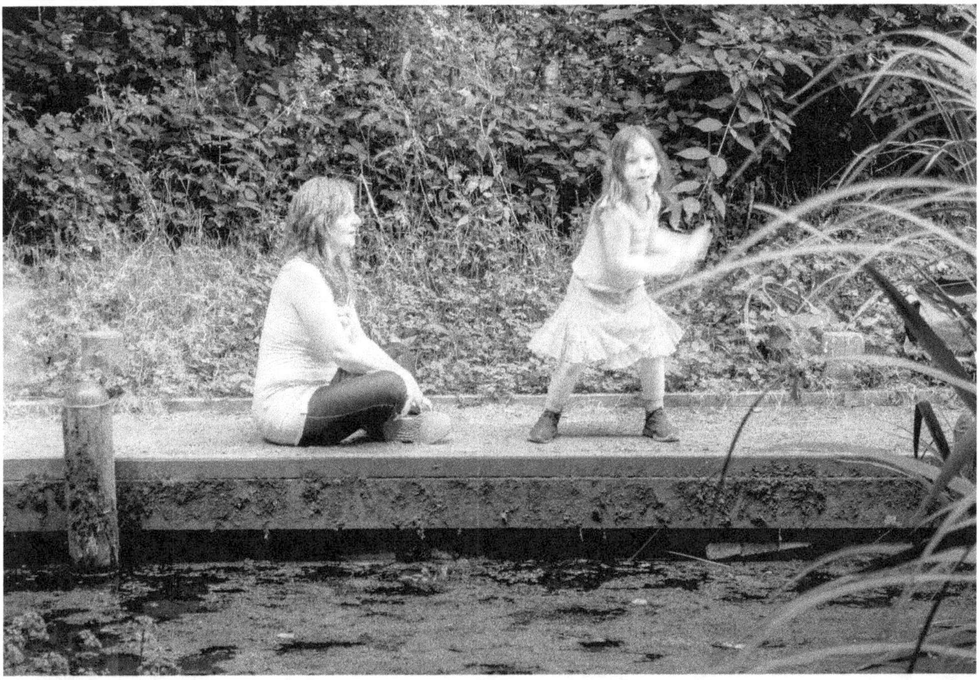

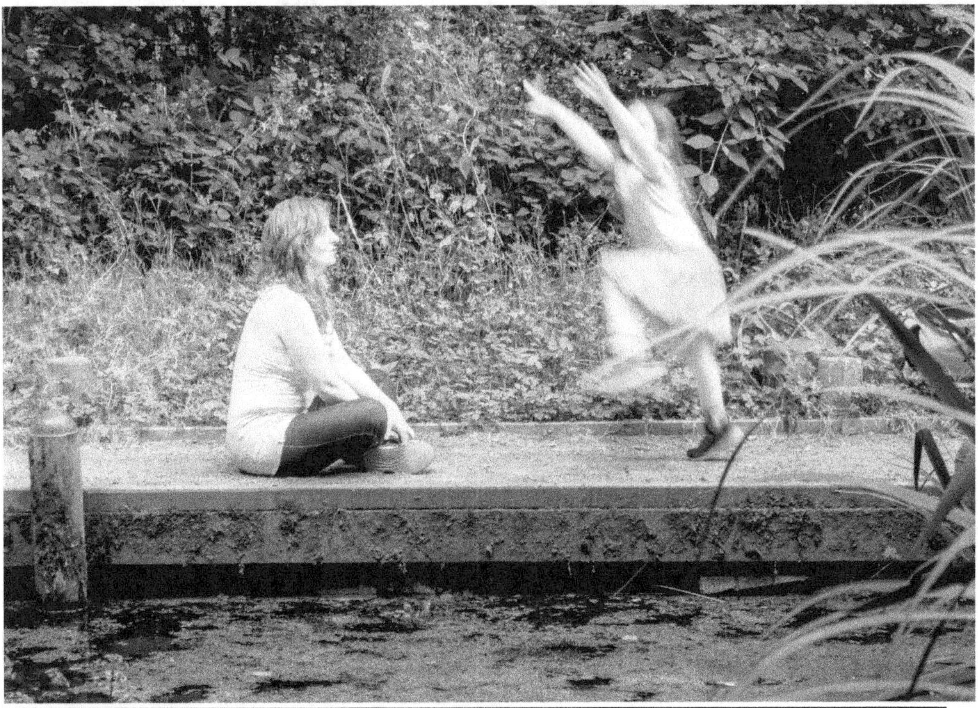

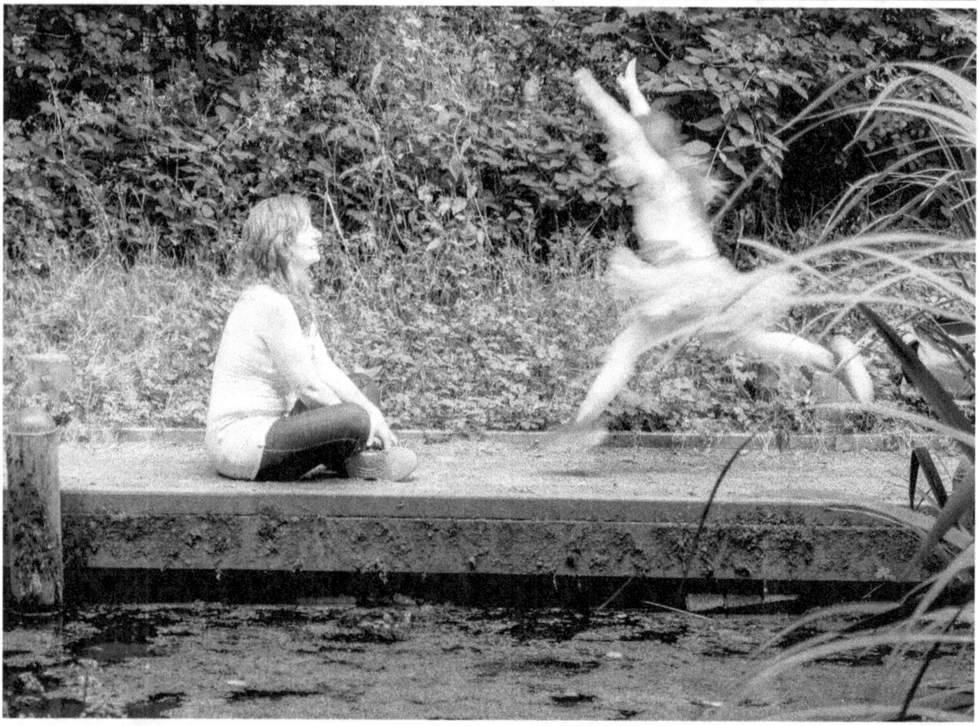

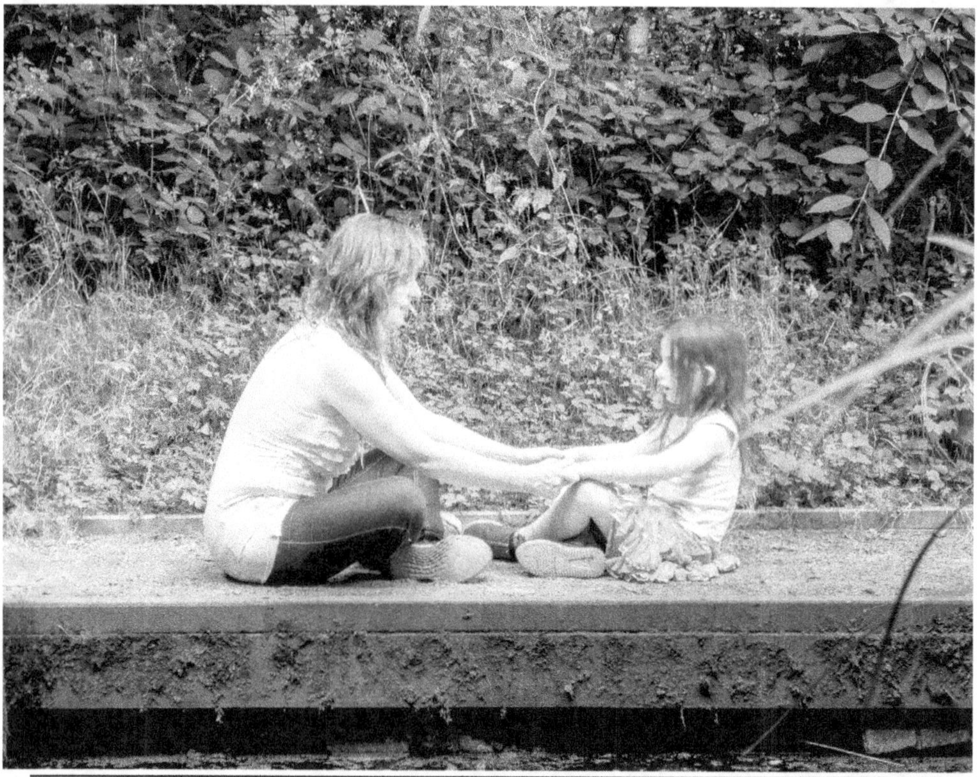

Your Spirit

Anxiety and stress affect all of us as one time or another but I can honestly say that the majority of carers that I have met suffer this to a degree that makes one wonder when they will breakdown.

The fifth activity is with the aim of connecting to through your energy system from the centre of your body and to experience your 'spirit come back to life'. To ground and liberate you and hopefully alleviate any anxieties that you may experience. Settle yourself in a place where you will not be disturbed for a good 10 to 15mins.

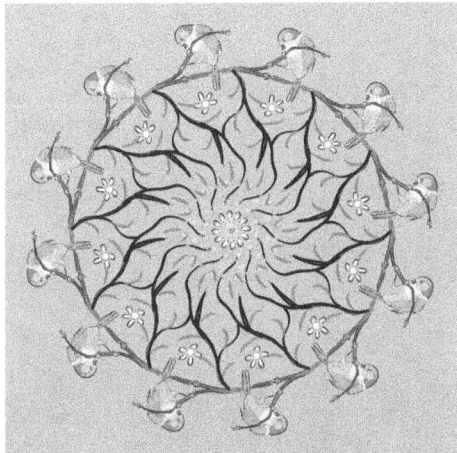

Bird - Pixabay by ID 1674061

- Start by taking a three or four rounds of breathing for the count of four, holding for the count of three; exhaling for the count of four and holding for three…REPEAT three more times. Really slowly down and telling yourself it is safe to let go into the chair/floor/cushion and allowing the restoring part of your central nervous system to move you!

- If you find yourself anxious and worrying about things turn your attention completely into focusing on the in breath and on the out breath.

- Focus your attention on the centre of your body and invite your spirit to be present by inwardly asking it. Breathe this invitation from your inner world and bring your attention and breathe to the base of your pelvis.

- In another moment from the base of the pelvis make a connection to the earth. Notice images, sense of space; colours, feelings etc. Keep breathing here and slow the connection to be made, taking the time you need.

- Next focus your attention and breathe into the crown of your head and from here into the space between you and the sky. Again, allow a connection to be made. Noticing what arises.

- Next, imagine the life giving energy of the earth and the sky flowing up from the earth and down from the sky into the centre of your body, just above the belly button and out.

- You are rooted and should feel your beautiful spirit flow through and around you. This energy is always available to you when you move this creativity through your centre.

Do feel less anxious? More settled into your skin?

Animal Dances

The sixth exercise is one to do with your child/client/friend. Using the images of Animals the 'animal dance' is lovely because you have so much fun.

- Choose which animal you want to explore today and find an appropriate piece of music for moving to. After a five minute warm up together and obviously feeling comfortable in the space you are using you are going to show a picture of the animal you are working with.

- Then you are going to play the music and together dance your animal.

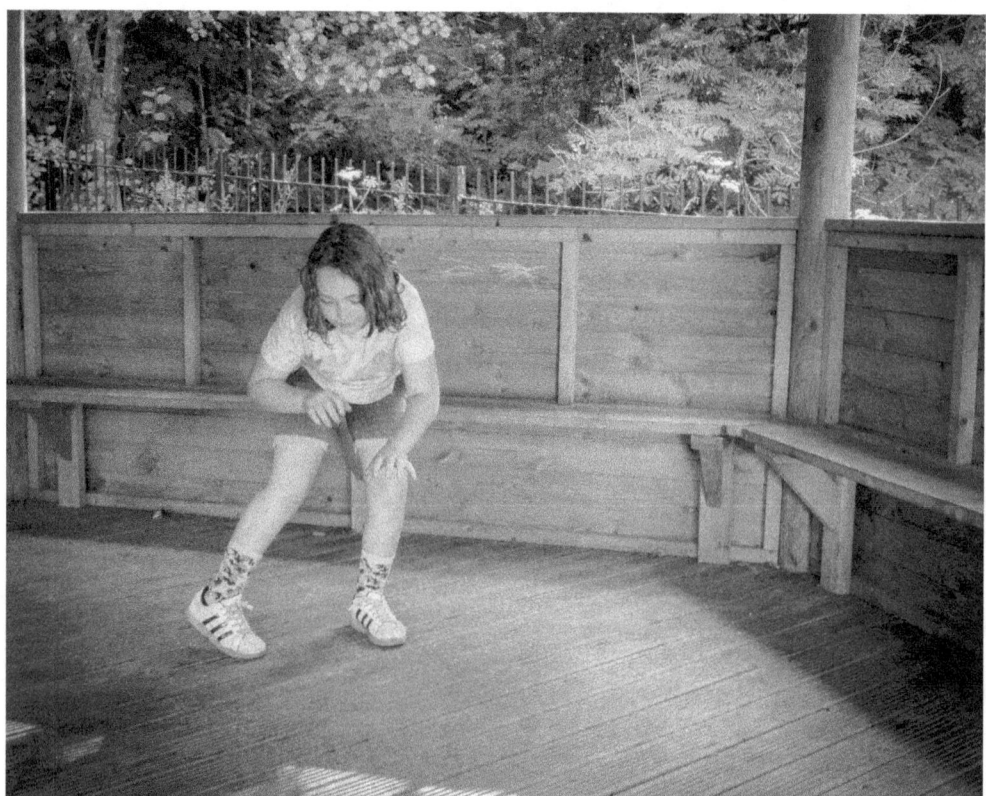

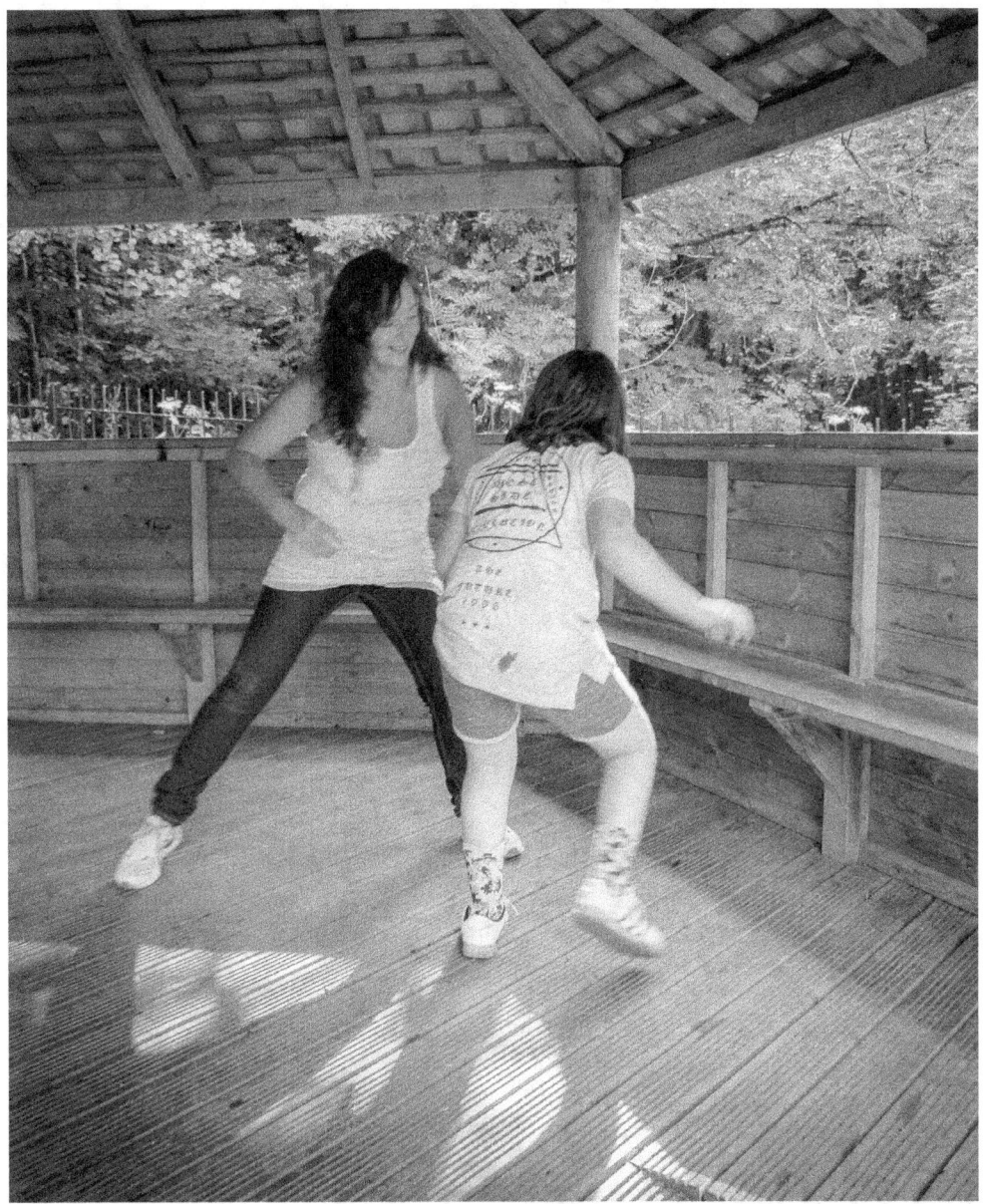

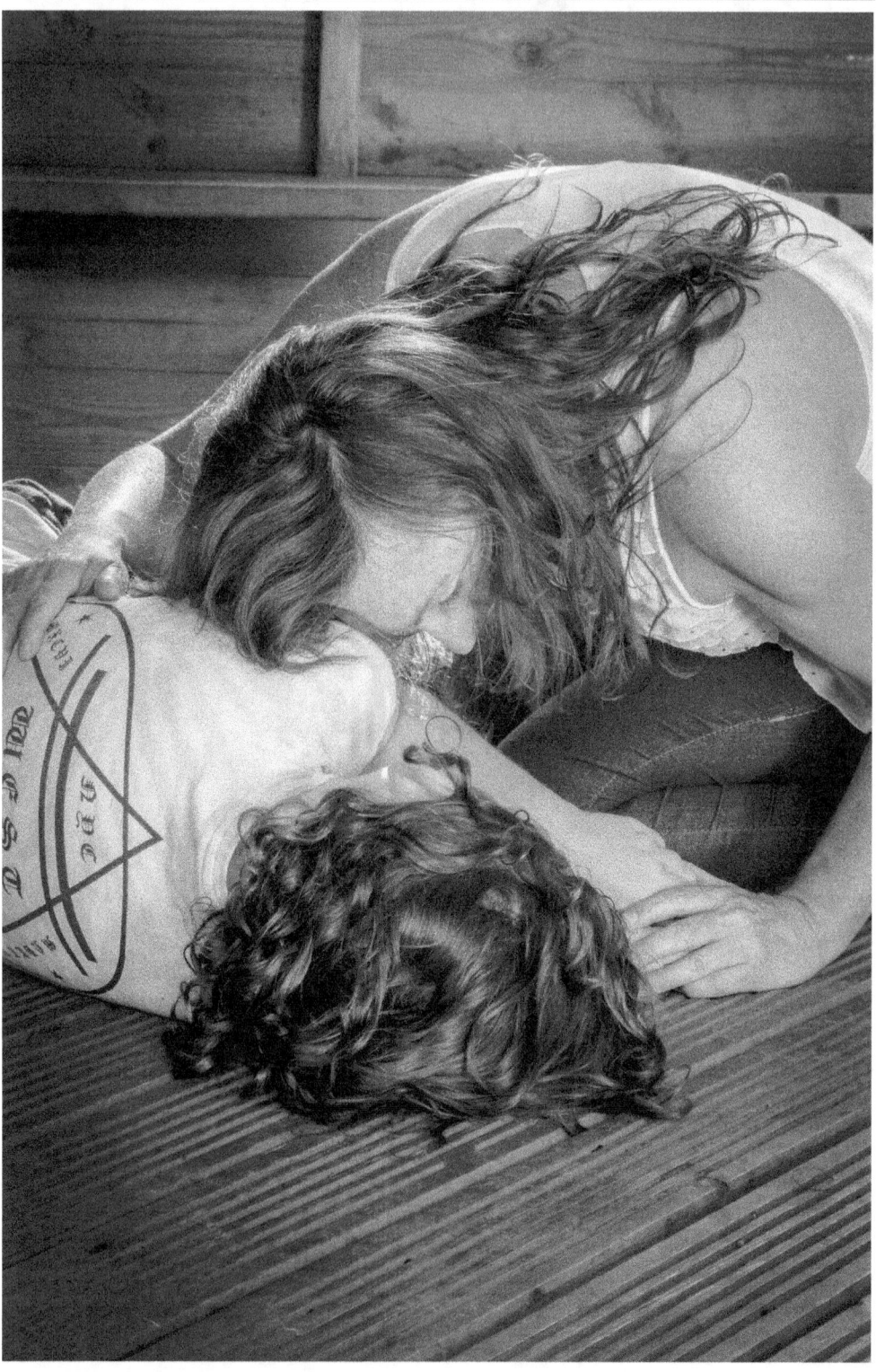

Karen Woodley - Movement Psychotherapy – RDMP

- Once the music has ended you are going to do the second stage which is the two animals dancing together with the idea of friendly play.

- The third step is where you as the leader are going to take care of the child with friendly, Warm and loving containment.

So connecting with the healthy energy and spontaneous movements is so vital for well-being because we are so conditioned into our roles and ways of being in order to fit into certain situations that we have lost that primitive bodily intelligence'. The vital energy of life that flows through our bodies if we allow it can be a real guiding light. At the same time the energy of sweetness and care is of fundamental importance and really is the only one we want to be communicating each and every day. This is what can save someone's life, help build strong immunity in our children and make this earth a better place.
So, with this in mind the last two exercises are designed for stimulating the vital energy and the sweet care of life.

Just dance!

Exercise seven 'Dance of integration' is for you alone to put your favourite track on and just dance and move your body without any worry of what others may think of you!

- You are going to be in a safe space alone and making sure you have a good ten minutes to just let your hair down.

- Be mindful of your chest, your hips and your head/neck as the idea is to let these parts of your body talk to each other!

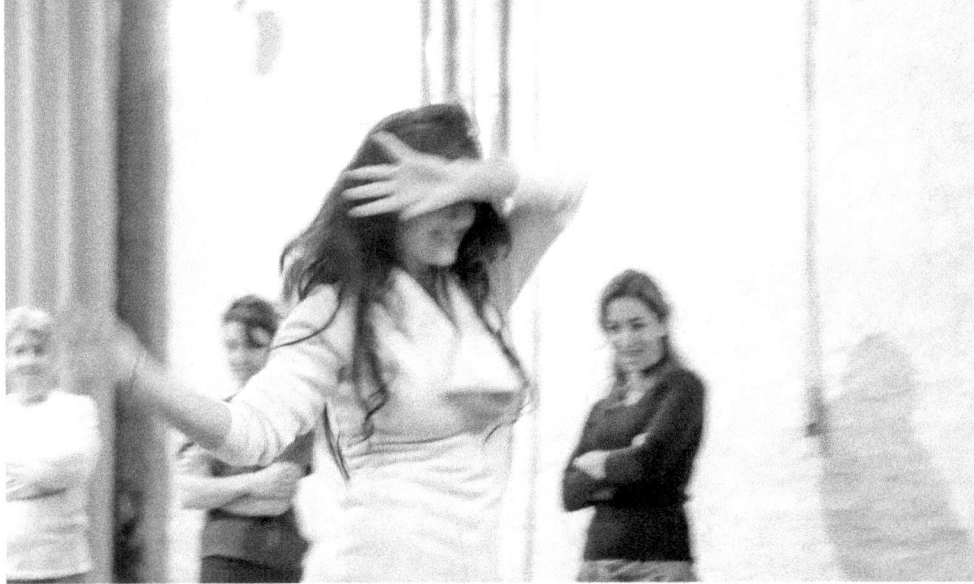

Give your light

Finally the last exercise 'Give your heart light' is to do with your child/client/friend and for this you will need:

- To be in a safe space and time where you will be undisturbed for a short while (the beauty of all these exercises is that you don't need to put by a whole lot of time in your day, they can fit in. Though you do need to be mindful of the preparation of yourself and for your child)

- To have the song "Unchained Melody" or similar.

- Have your child stand (or if this is not possible, placed) in front of you with their eyes closed if they are comfortable with this.

- Place your hands on your heart and invite your beautiful inner light, with your eyes closed invite this light from your heart to expand and with your hands you are going to bring this from your heart into your cupped hands, like a warm glowing fire.

- In honour of and with the deepest reverence and love for who you have in front of you you are going to baptise them with this light.

- Start at the top of their head and very slowly pull this light down to their toes, taking all the time in the world!

- With your committed attention and direct intention to shower them with light with an attitude of gratitude for their humanity and what they give each day you will root them into a space of love.

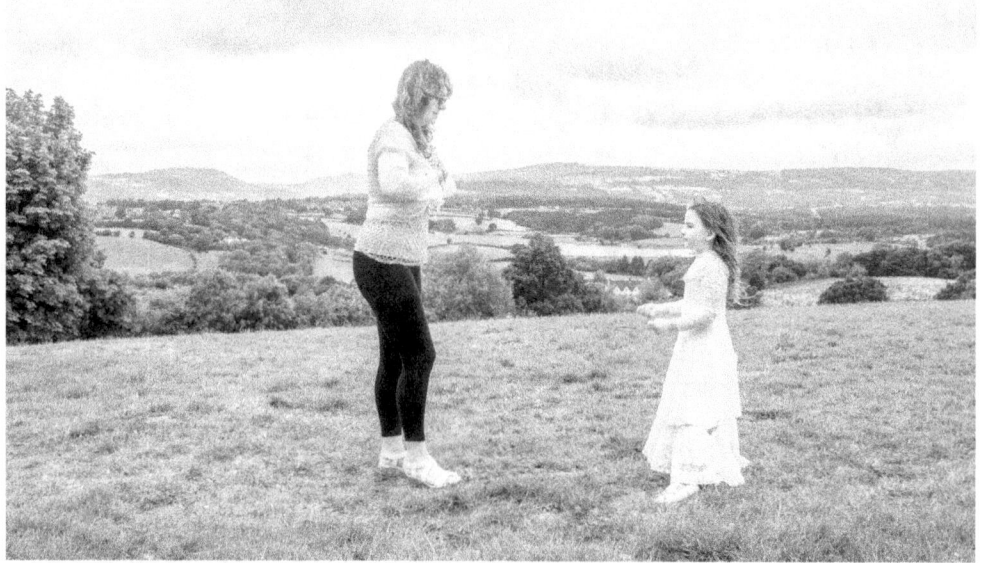

Karen Woodley - Movement Psychotherapy – RDMP

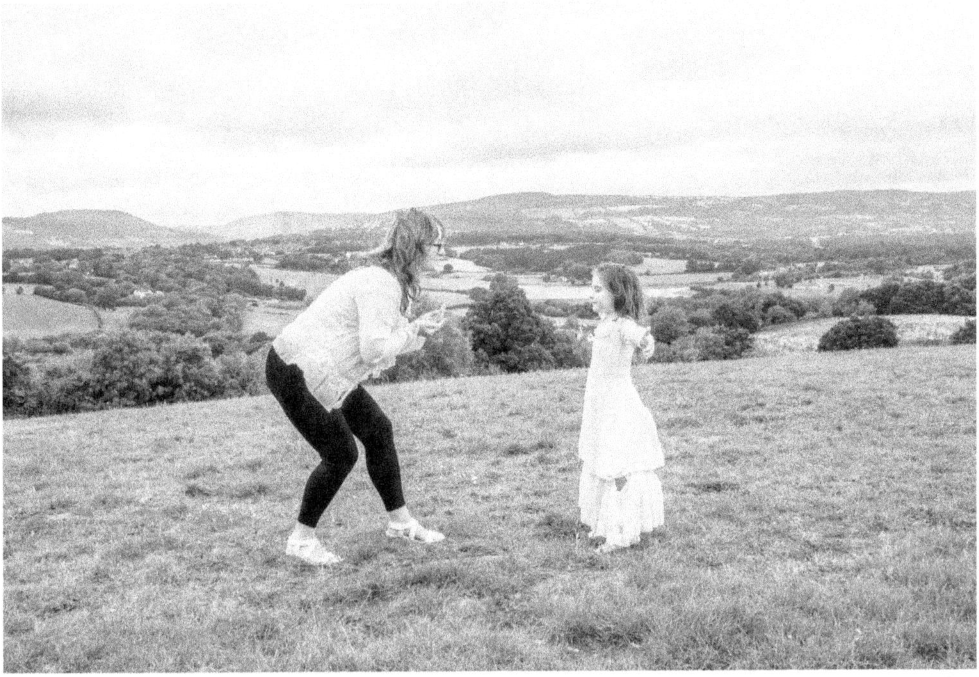

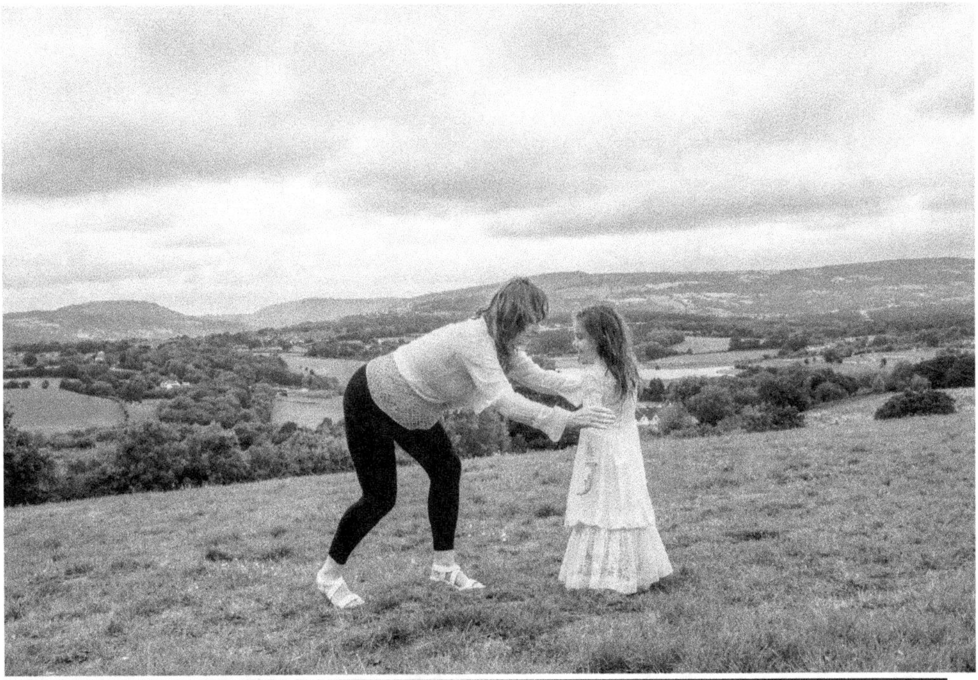

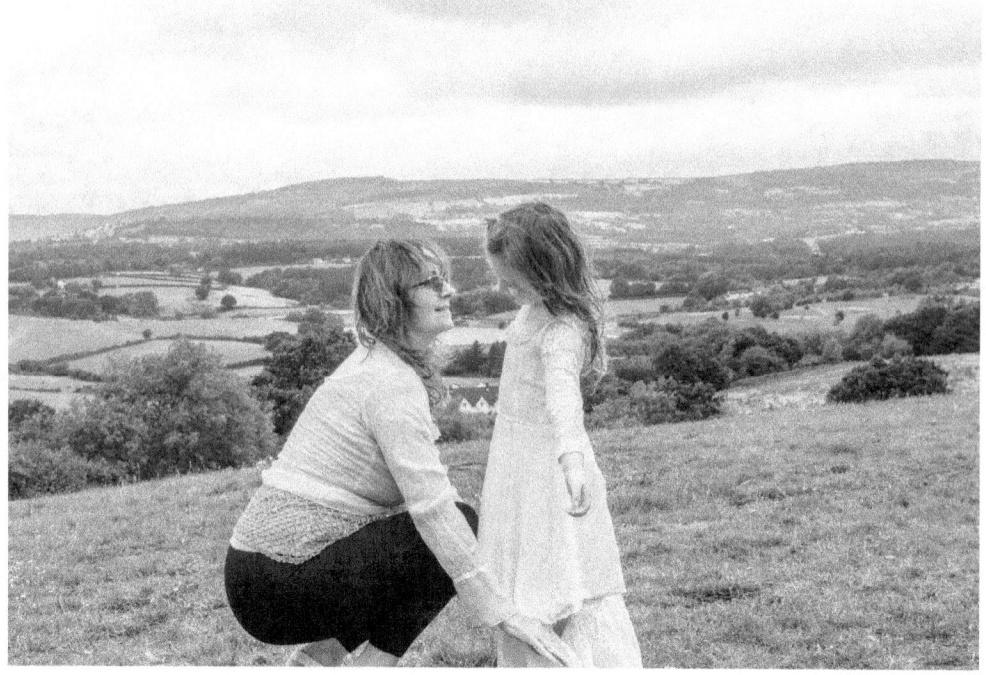

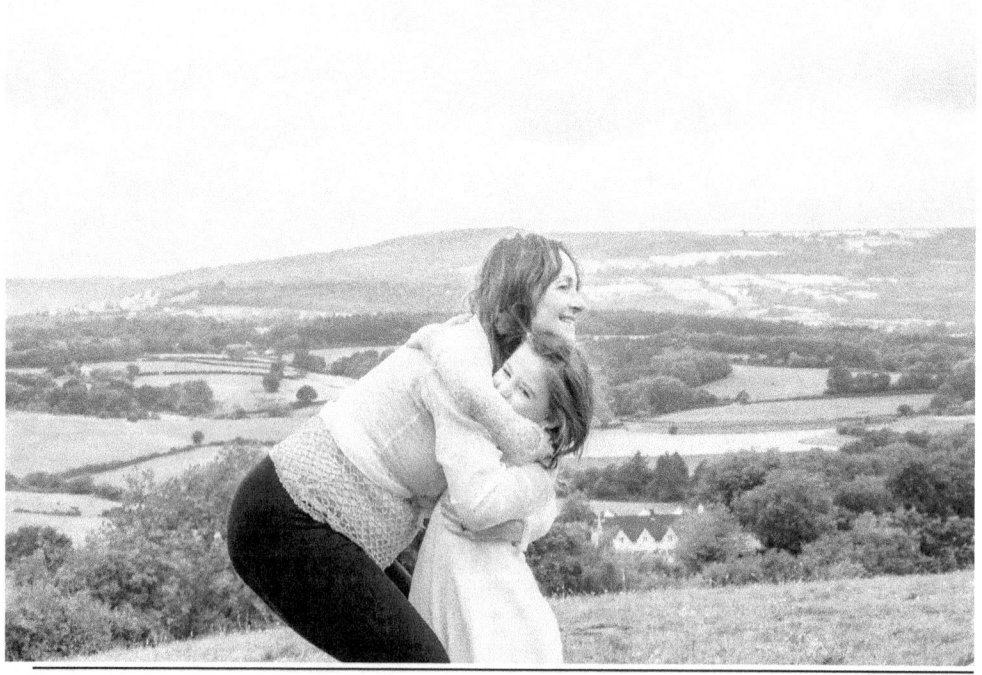

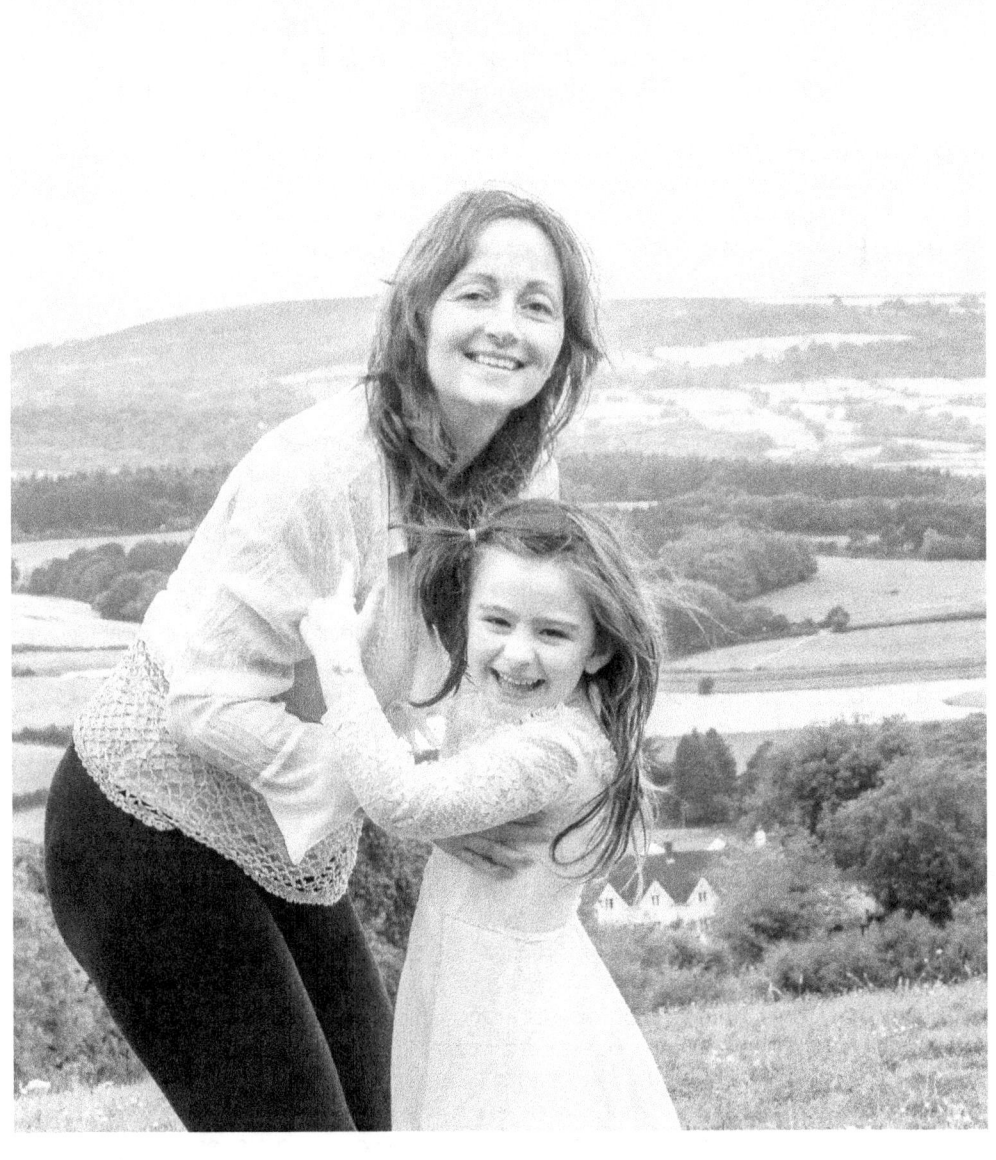

Putting life in the centre and Ideas for adding a little love and restoration at home

The true person centred, humanistic therapeutic approach comes from the work of (Rogers, 2003). And the way I like to explain it is that we simply want to connect and commune with the life force and unique source of energy that flows through each person; it is the life force within that just thrives under loving conditions. Love is what makes the world go round!!! A sound corny but, it is like this.

> *"What we call the secret of happiness is no more a secret than our willingness to choose life"*
> *Leo Buscaglia*

As a carer you well know that the 'person centred' care plan is at the heart of everything you do and in a way this booklet is a guide to help you go a little deeper into what it means to be person centred and how it feels when you start to work with things like Honesty, Acceptance; Respect and Compassion

Being honest starts with you honestly being the feelings and emotions that are flowing through you and not just pleasing others all the time because sooner or later you will burn out!.

So, what does it mean to be honest with your feelings? It means listening to your body, noticing the gentle nudges of hunger, of need for rest; for acceptance, to be understood; the need for air and intimacy etc. (© 2005 by Center for Non-violent Communication) and actually honouring those needs. Are you honest with yourself and others every day?

Accepting without judgement with the understanding that we all do the best we can do. Do you judge / or are you harsh with yourself or others?
With somebody you are caring for it is about embracing them wholeheartedly and when you hit a wall of 'not liking something about them' and especially because your role is to care, you find a way to overcome this egocentric way and you open your heart even more.

So, how can we do this? By respecting who they are and how they are through unconditional love, which is not the same as personal love. It is bigger and wider and we can all do it. And, what's more if your profession is that of a 'Carer', you have a duty to do it. I remember when my Grandfather was sick and he had to have a carer come into his home to look after him at mealtimes and things like this how I would pray that the person was real and with a kind heart offering light along the way because this is what he deserved and, without this light that shone through in each encounter of smiles, of taking time to listen; of eating together etc. the dignity of life is not respected and we do a disservice to humanity.
So, how do you love yourself and others? People do not need clever words or special degrees in this or that they just need a loving person to hold everything

that they are. The simplest, gentlest, sweetest thing in the world and it all takes a moment. If you find this within yourself you will find it in others. Being Compassionate is not only to feel the feelings of another but to do something about it!

I think if we have a deep respect for human life, our own and that of the people we care for then we not only help light the forces of 'life' within them and ourselves but we are somehow acknowledging that with the right connection, communication and care everyday can be joyful. The reason why you are a carer is because you care. Giving person centred care really encompasses knowing what the person likes to do, who is important to them in their life; If music helps them to be happy, what makes them have good energy all of these things.

Some exercises and ideas to use at home together that can help to awaken the beautiful inner light of your heart

(In this section please make sure that you ensure you have a safe, quiet space and unrushed time enough for working through the exercises carefully. Centre yourself and see each one as sacred time)

Sometimes at home it could be that you need a little help in helping to soothe and relax your child/client/friend and so this chapter is specifically with this in mind. Again though the first exercise is for you and can be part of your new self-care regime and the second exercise is one you can introduce at home.

Connection

How do you connect with yourself and others? Do you take care of yourself and do nice things for yourself? For example have nice warm towels ready for you after a bath, use nice smelling perfumes or take 5 mins in the middle of a busy day to just tune into your breath and imagine a rainbow ball of light wash you from the crown

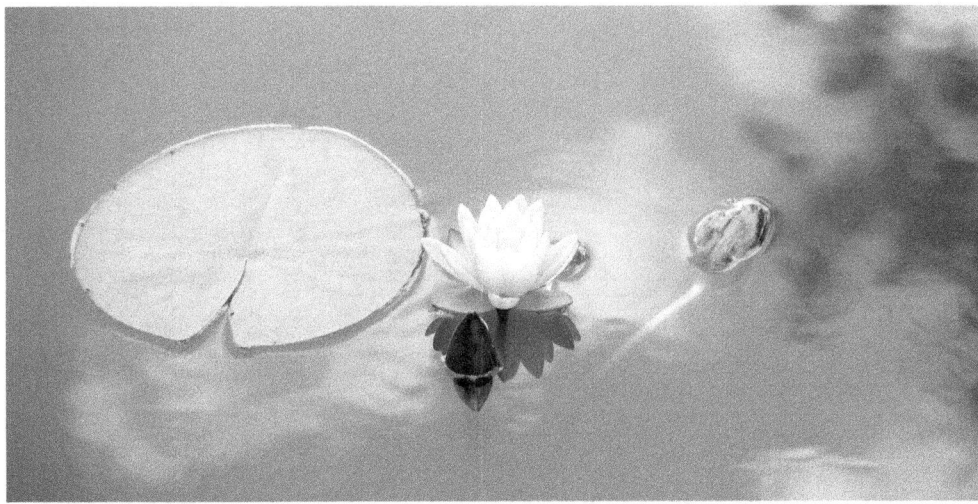

of your head to the bottoms of your feet. With others, do you connect from your heart each time or are you connecting with your stress and problems and heavy energies?

- Exercise one: "The inner-fire" - place your hands on your heart whilst playing a beautiful piece of music. Both hands on your heart and place your chin to your chest. In this intimate connection with yourself let's do a 'dance of inner connection'. Feel into your heart and ask yourself / notice how you are feeling, what is in your heart. Notice this truth inside of you. As you are breathing with your hands on heart allow this connection with your hearts gentle voice to move you. The chinese say the heart is fire, what is your fire telling you? At the end of 3 or 4 mins you can end this posture and come back to where you are and what is around you.

- Exercise two: 'Playing ball' this simple game is one you can do at home to focus in a fun way to build a more present and light-hearted connection with your child / client.
  Find a good, safe space to use and perhaps play your child's favourite music
  Simply throwing and catching the ball back and forth

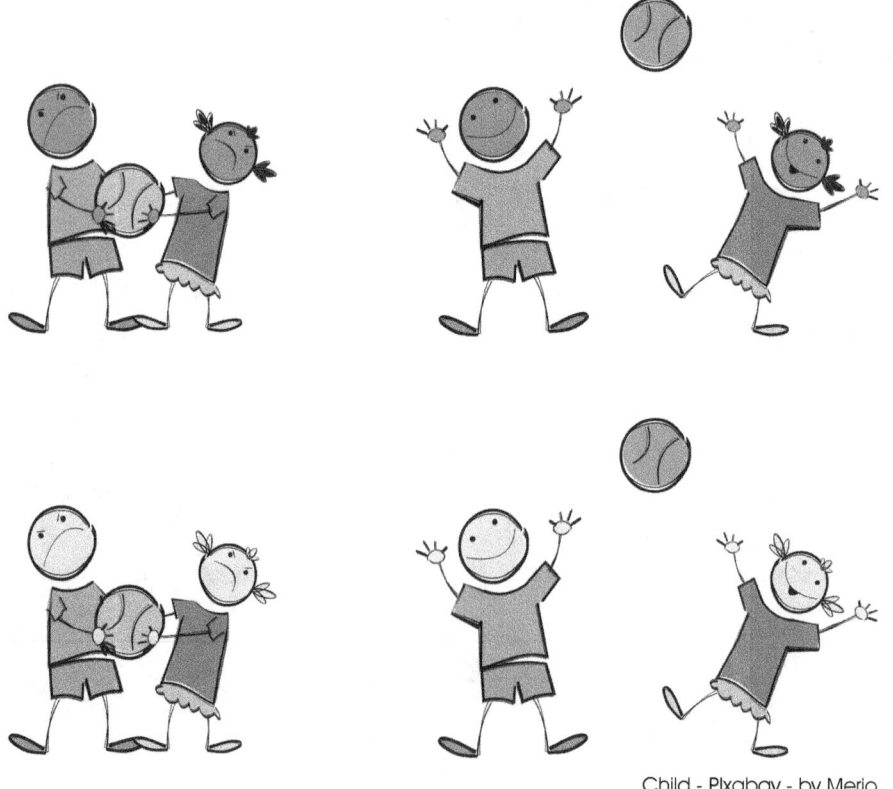

Child - Pixabay - by Merio

Could be rolling / could be using words each time you catch it like for example blue and then your child says red (or not)
Five or ten minutes of this game with focused attention is enough to start a lovely connection

A communication key

Communication – do you communicate your needs easily? Do you find this hard? Do you communicate gentleness care and kindness or do you communicate information and 'intelligent knowledge' that may be useful to people but will not let them know you understand them for example? When chimpanzees approach each other they show their hands to show they are friendly and want to communicate and connect. They speak with their hands!

- Exercise one: 'Your Hands' Again play a beautiful piece of music if you so wish, starting with placing your awareness and focus on your hands, put them out in front of you and begin to appreciate them Okay, after a minute or so of centering yourself in your awareness here you are going to offer your hands to the world and notice what this is like for you. Allow your hands to move in ways where they are connecting with the world, receiving the world...what is like? When you feel you have your hands and their experience in the world, remember that they that are in the direct line of your heart, the same energy circuit of your heart, you are going to place them over your face and really appreciate your face, breathing in the energy from your hands to your face.

  NOTE: it is important to let go of all guilt, blame and criticism to yourself, let it go and connect with the appreciation and tender affection directed towards yourself.

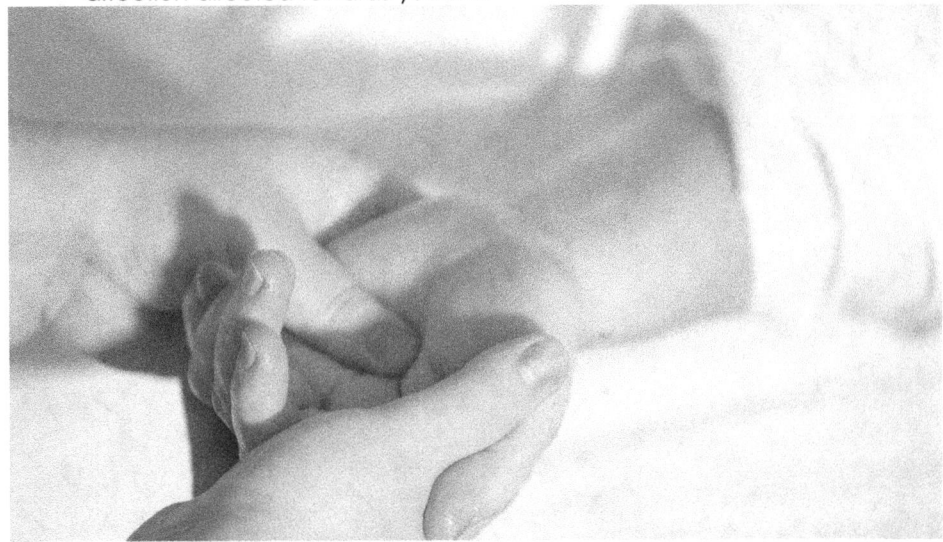

Treatment - Pixabay by Andreas160578

After doing this for a couple of minutes or so you are going to place your hands on your heart centre and feel in to your unique heart, what is this like for you?
Then you are going to move to you belly.
A moving meditation where you pour appreciation, gratitude and love in-towards yourself.

- Exercise two: 'Friendly Fuzziness': You are going to play a nice piece of music and focusing on your hands you are going to offer them to your child. Imagine that you cannot speak or hear anything and approach your child/client from a distance and slowly communicate a message of wanting to communicate with them and understand who they are. As you approach you are going to reach out to communicate 'friendly fuzziness' offering your hands for them to accept or not. If they accept then gently and sweetly caress their hands and continue this for as long as they allow. If they reject your offer then introduce a soft toy and start to explore the tactile sensation of this together

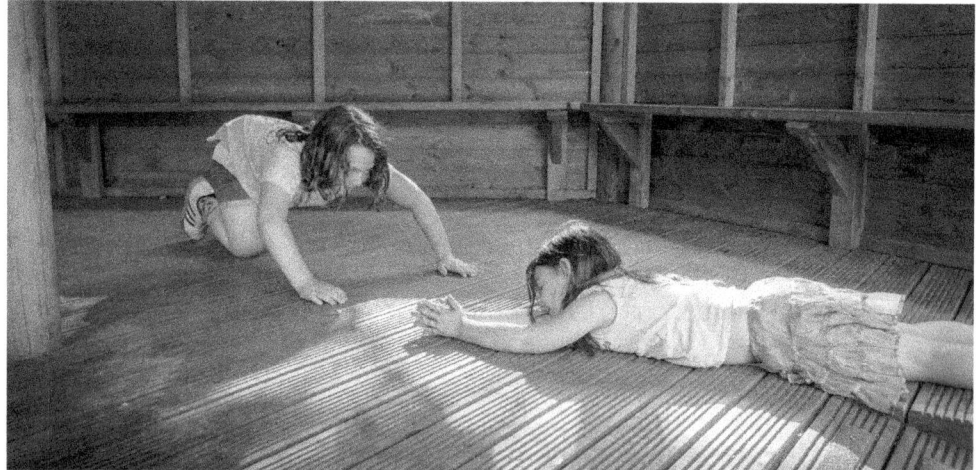

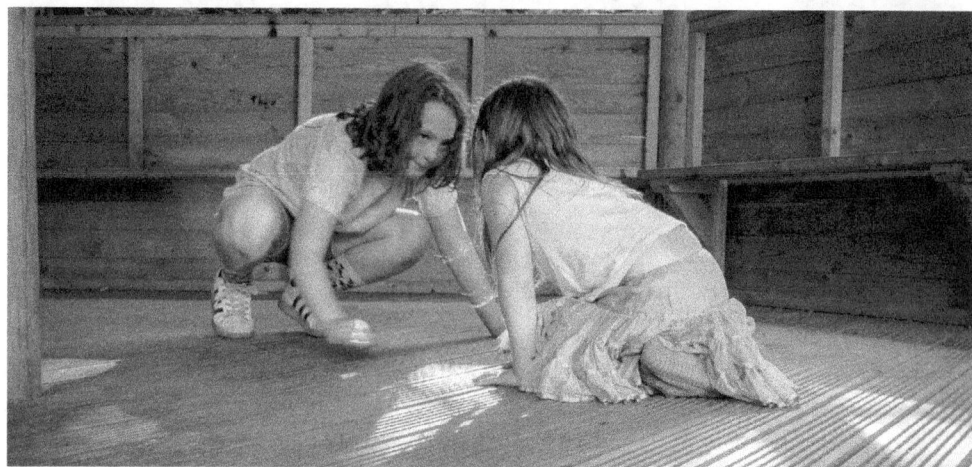

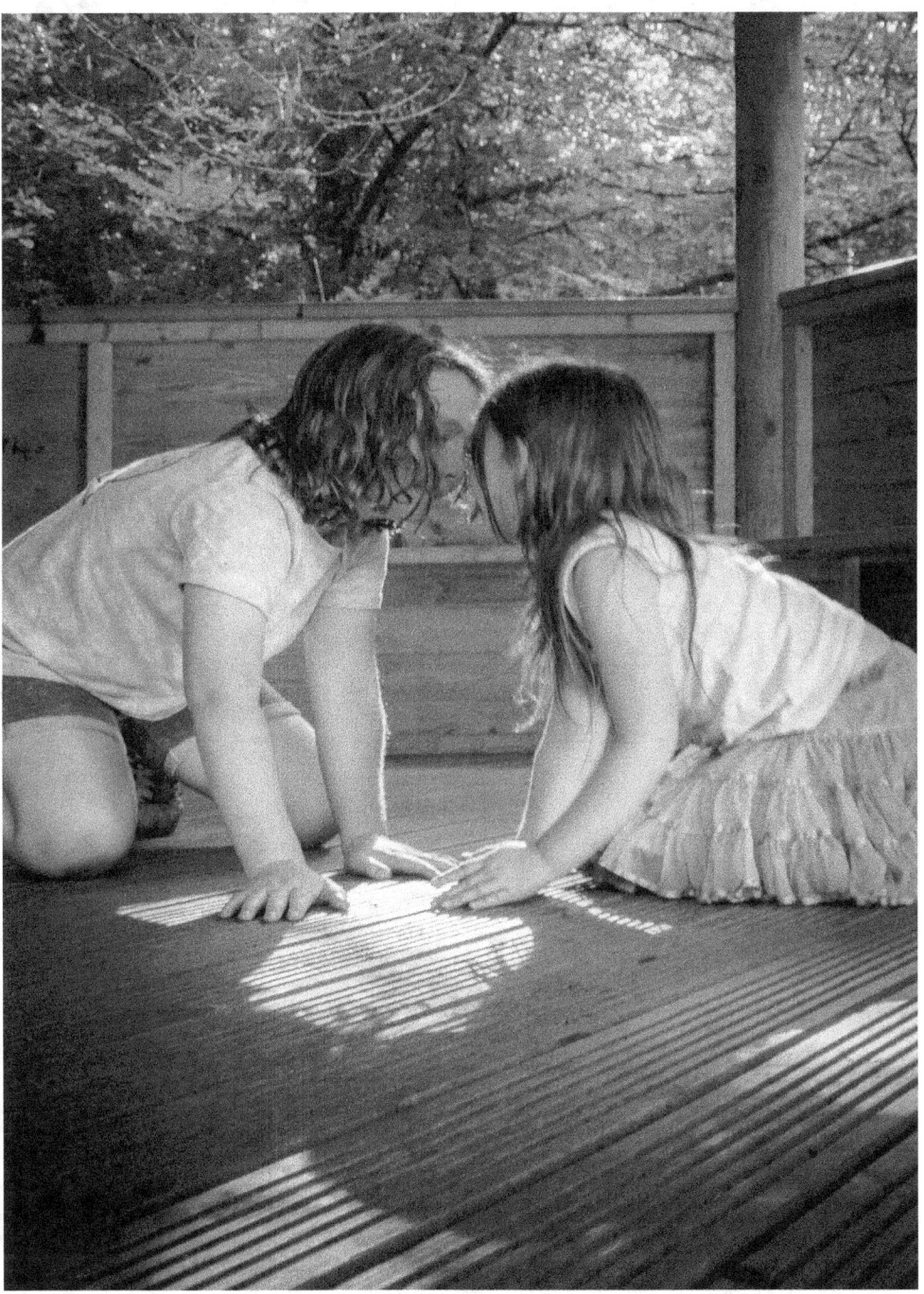

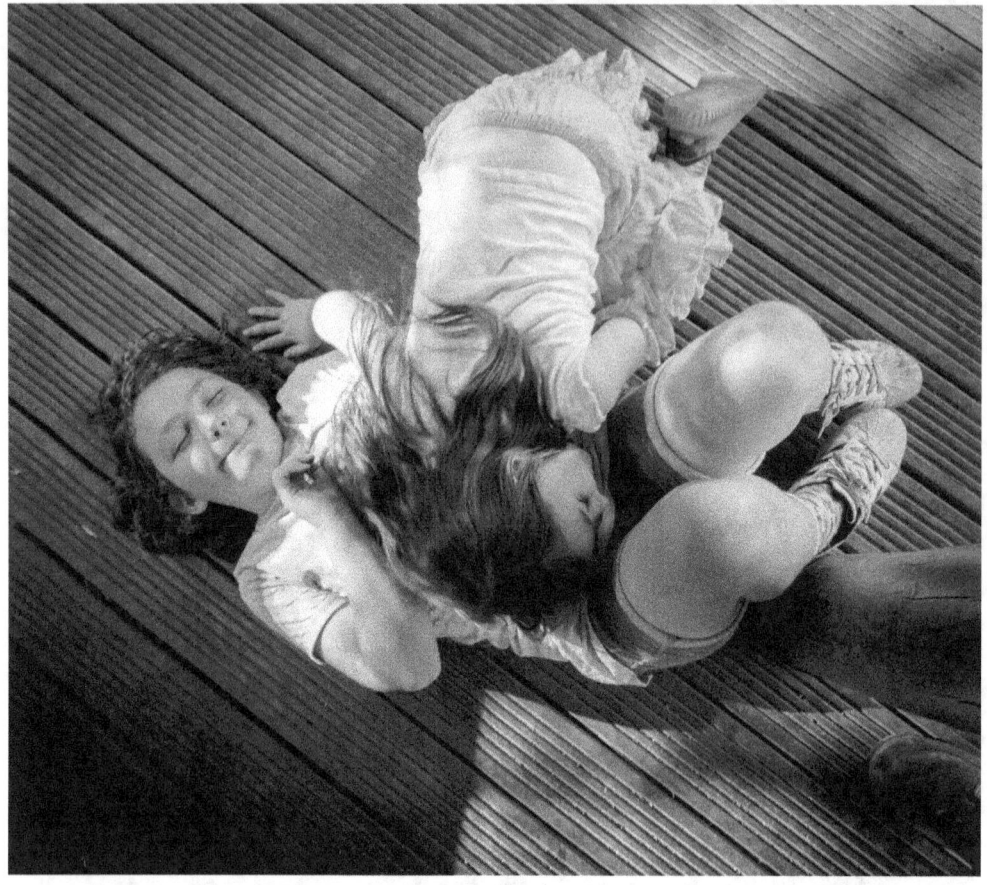

Affection

Care – What does it mean to care to you? Do you allow people to care for you? Do you take good care of yourself, listening to and honouring your own needs or do you get carried away with the strain and stresses of survival? Affection is a higher evolutionary state that is not necessarily linked with being sensitive or intelligent. It is a feeling of love for humanity.

Exercise one: 'Rocking the baby'

- Using soft music and having your partner sit over your lap

- You will need to be seated on the floor with the back propped up

- You partner sits with their hips touching your hips and facing you

- Then leaning into you as you hold them as you would a baby

- Holding them and looking into their eyes with the eyes that come from the sweet fire of your heart

- Stay until the end of the track and then with a hug you can end this exercise

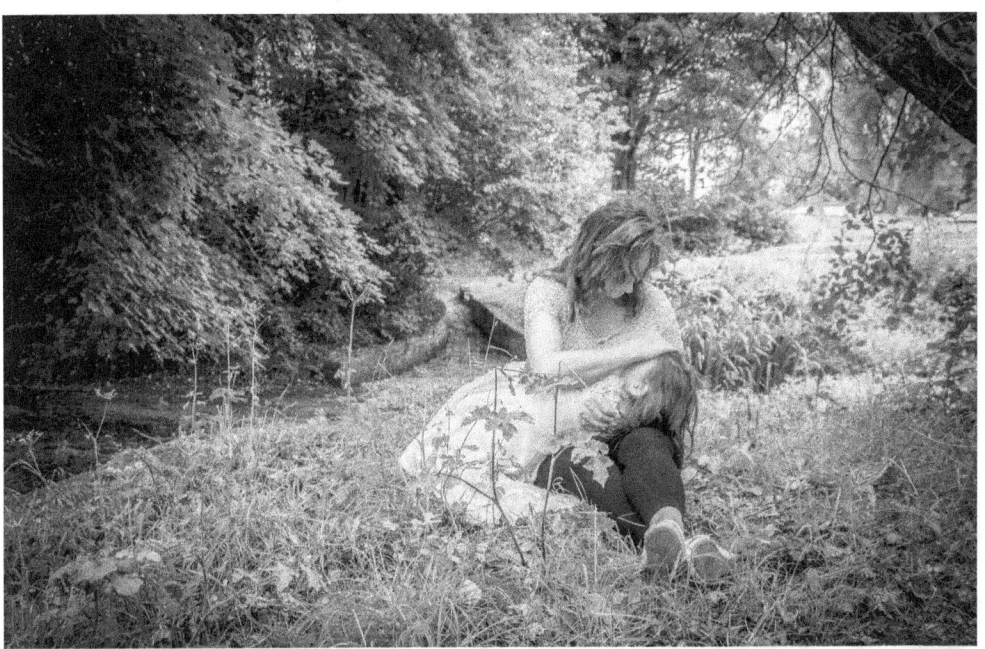

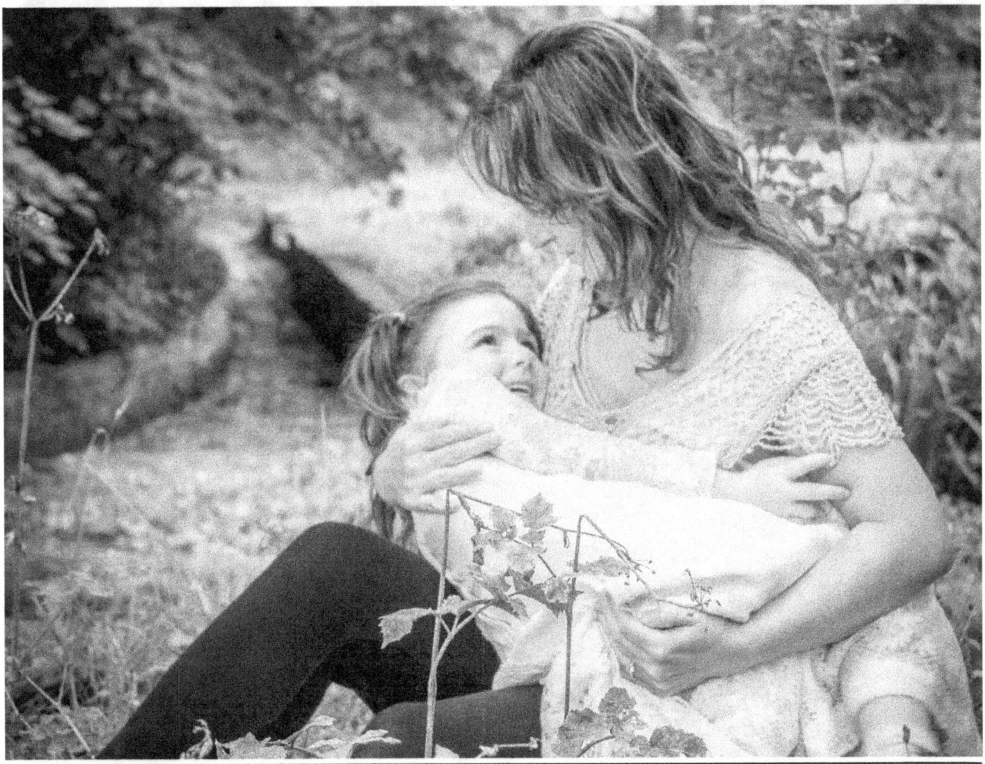

Exercise two: 'Breathing together'

- Again using appropriate music and either sitting directly behind your partner with your legs wrapped around them allowing them to put their head back on your chest or standing and holding them in your embrace

- Connecting to the breath and resting your head on their shoulder

- Encourage them to do the same

- Like two beautiful baby chicks or birds resting and breathing without forcing anything

- Allow the music to come to an end and then come out of this.

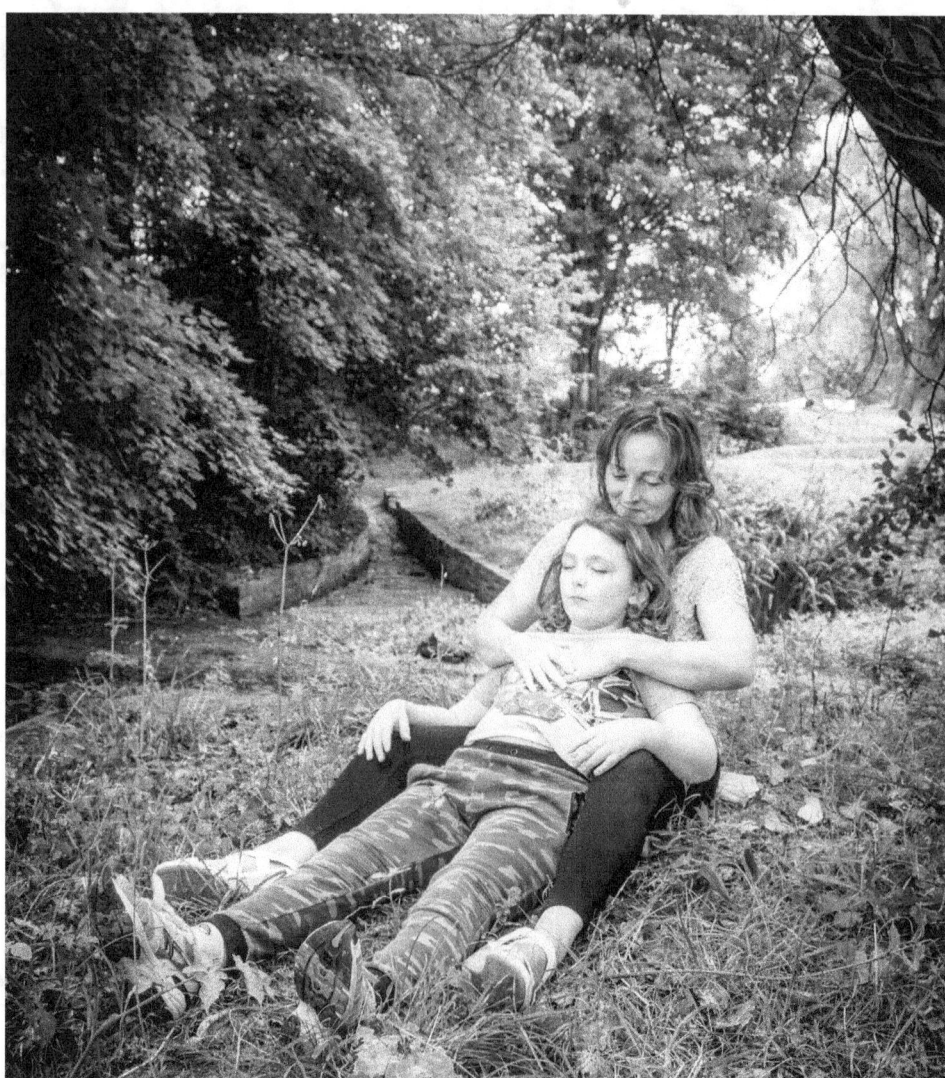

Exercise three: 'Caress of the hair'

- Either sitting cross legged and opposite your partner or standing directly in front of them

- With lovely music playing you place your hands on your heart and connect with your heart light

- Ask your partner to close their eyes and just rest their hands in their lap

- When you are ready you are going to take out your heart light and from the centre of your hands soft and shaped like your heart place them on your child's hair

- Slowly and with dedication you are going to stroke/caress the hair from the top to the bottom. Delicately, sensitively and with all the care and love you can to give containment and the presence of a containing and healing guide.

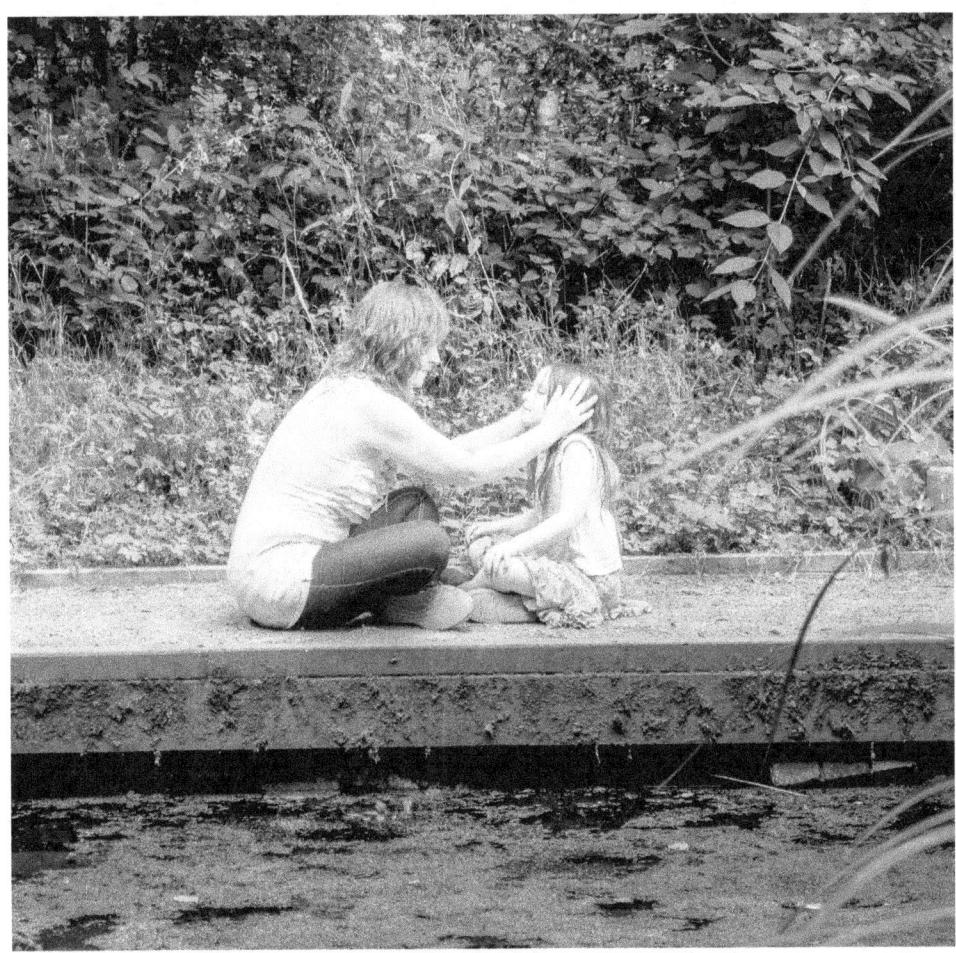

Exercise four: 'Paint with light'

- Have your partner lay down in a comfortable position

- Tell them you are going to paint their face with different coloured light

- Invite this light to flow from your heart to your hands

- Use it to paint your partner.

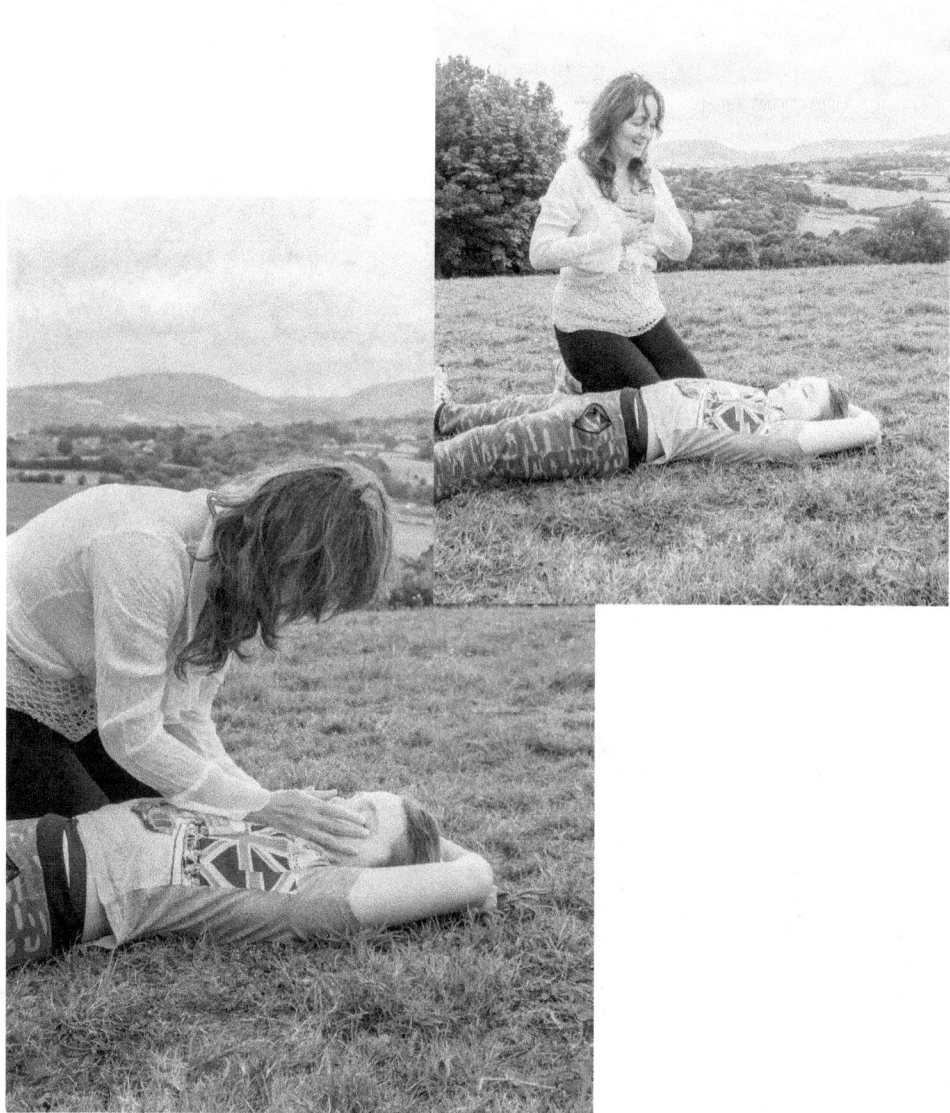

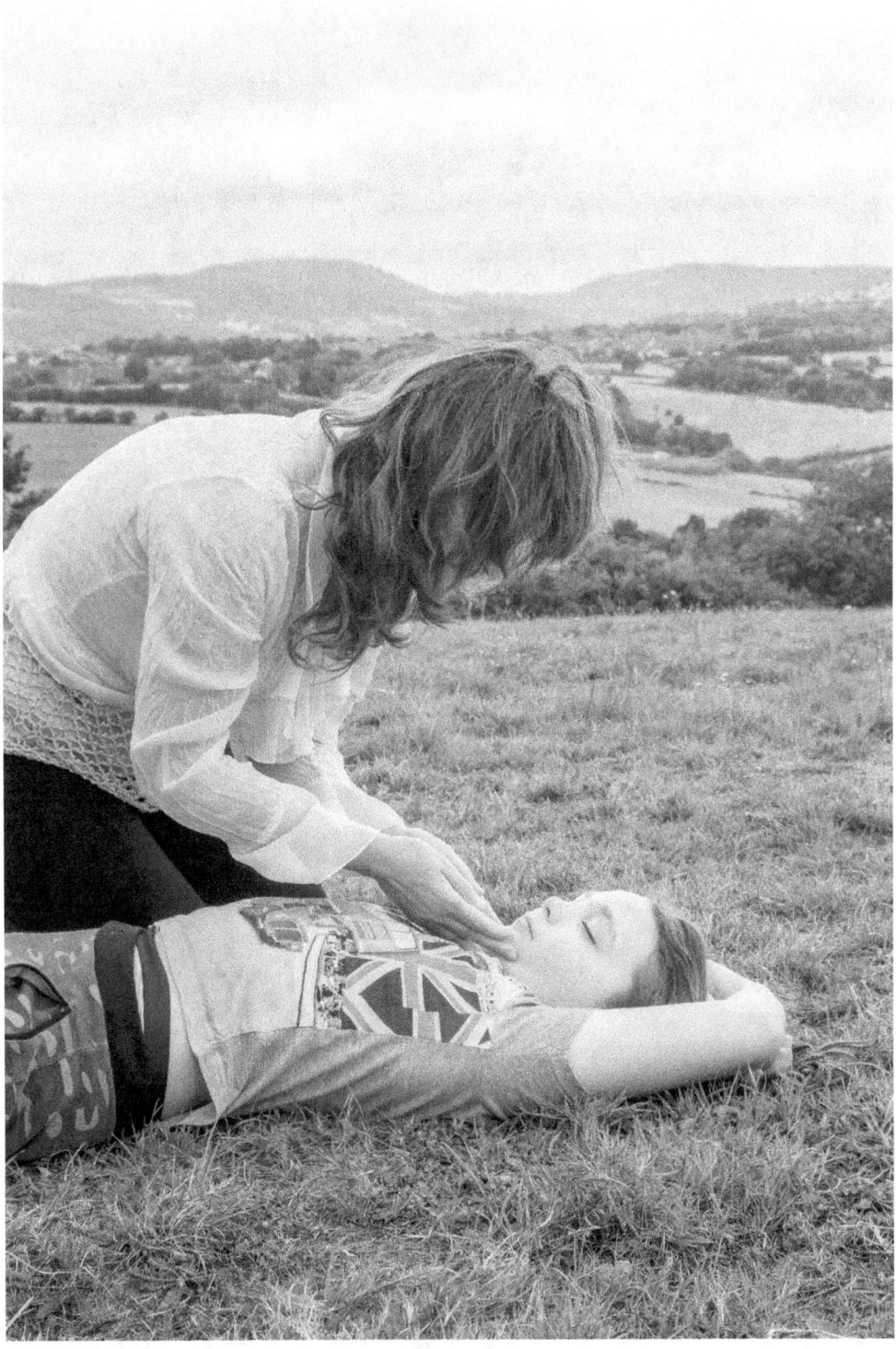

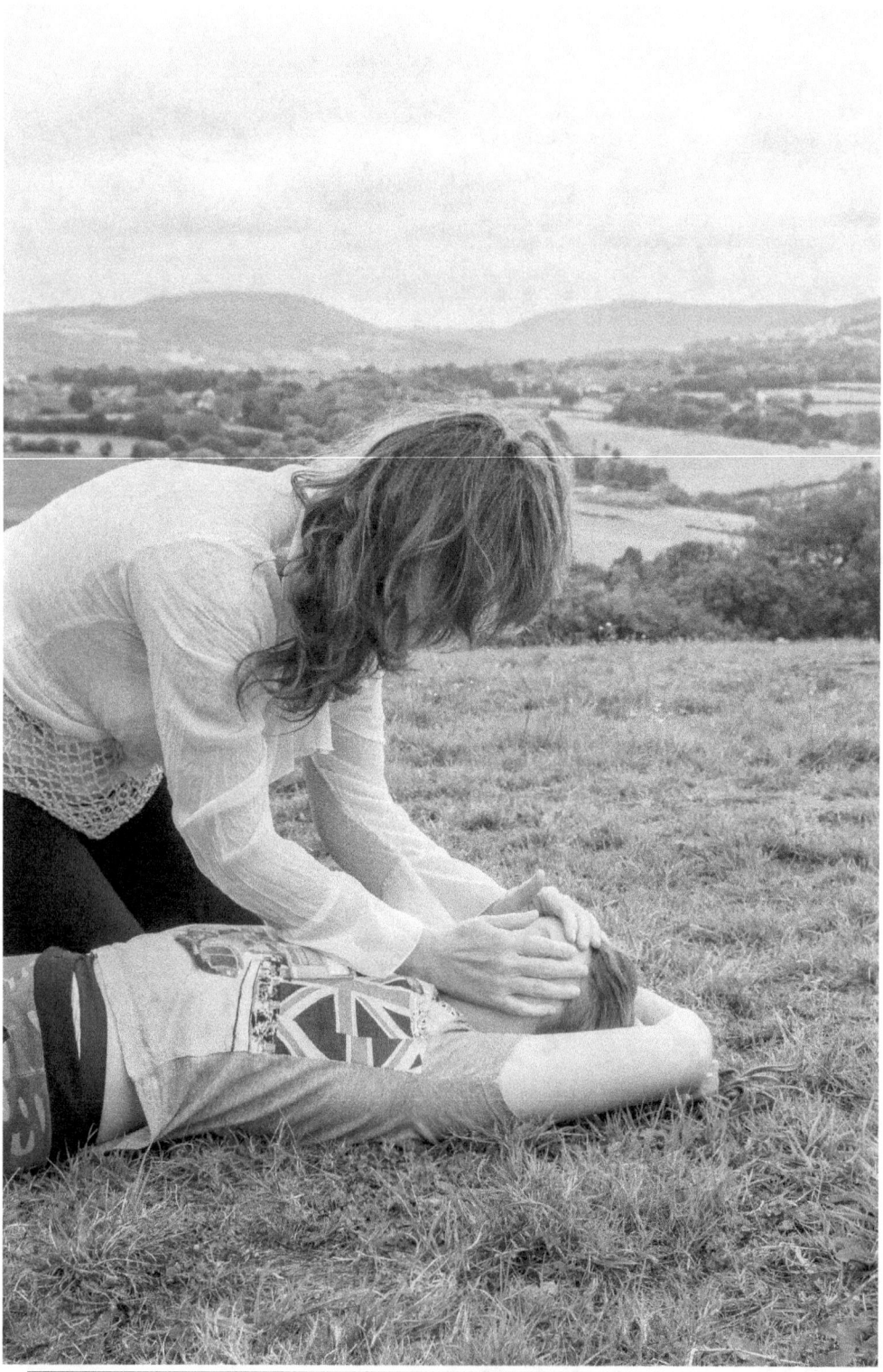

PART THREE

Colourful Notes

In this chapter of the book I share some stories with you that have touched me over the years and inspired me to write this companion book.

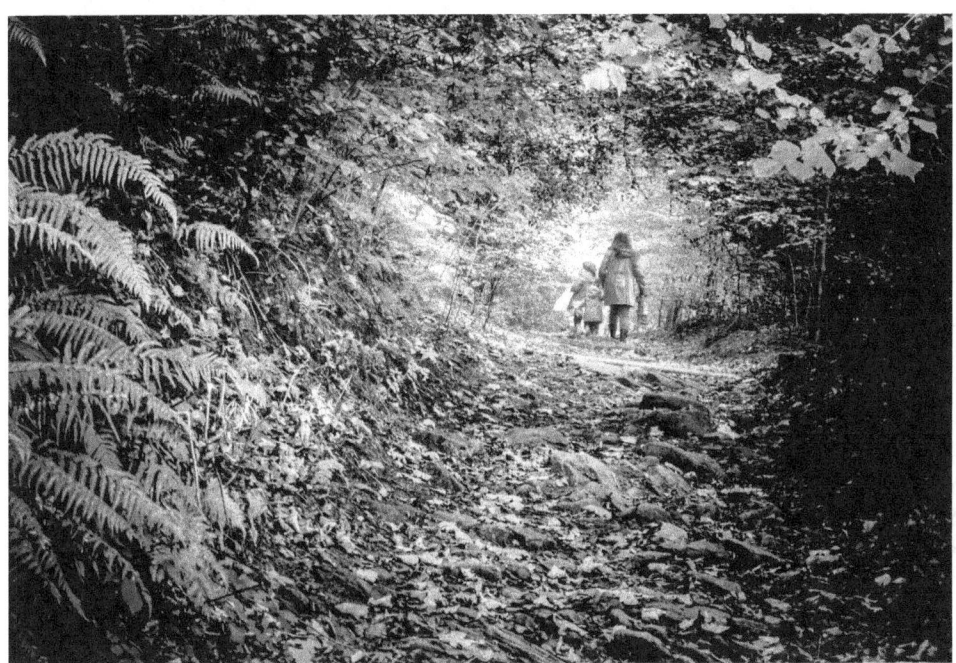

Mimi and her family

Mimi came along for sessions at the organisation where I have worked for a good ten years in all. She came as a little baby with her mum and dad and also with some family support workers from a deaf blind charity, Sense Cymru.

This little girl, so beautiful loved making music and the playful movement part of the sessions. She was so adored by her parents who had not slept for almost two years!

She had charge syndrome and as a result would never roll onto her belly. Knowing that the belly is the bodies centre and a point from which to become centred and begin movement from we would encourage this as she roamed around the space.

One day the grandmother approached me and told me that she was so concerned for Mimi's parents and that she thought if they were not able to get some kind of help soon she was afraid that the family unit would just crumble.

This really shook me. I suppose it was something to do with a little girl, so alive and vital in her spirit with a disability that involves so many invasive medical procedures and physical difficulties that I wondered if she felt terror at not really having an earthed compass in her body from which to be guided by! On top of this her parents were adorably kind-hearted and young too.

As this grandmother was speaking to me I had an idea along with my colleagues to create a pamper sessions for mums and dads as a way to offer a little respite. Even if it were to open a space for mum and dad to experience for a moment how they need to care for themselves along the way, for without caring for them they will run out of the energy needed for their child. As it transpired the family never got along to the parent session but in their honour they are running to this day!

George and family

George Started coming along to me for sessions from a little one year old diagnosed with Downs Syndrome with his mum who was so very emotional with her situation. She was told by the doctor that her little boy would never walk and talk and as you might imagine this turned her world upside down!

Deep down inside I think she felt guilty. My heart went out to her as she was such a lovely lady who adored her son and was, understandably, having such difficulty time facing things. They would come into sessions and when they would leave I always felt 'God, there must be some way to really help' mum short of pampering her as much as I could when she was in session!

Children born with Down's syndrome have 1 extra gene than the rest of us, an extra chromosome 21 material in their cells....it should be called Up's syndrome! Perhaps the only real help is when somebody realises that they must care for themselves. Be honest about their needs and find simple daily life ways to do this!

Glenda and mum

Glenda has been coming in to sessions for a good eight years now. Every week she joins her friends in her group; mum comes along with the carer too. She is a young woman who does not have speech and I think her diagnose is 'Angel Syndrome', such apt and lovely names!

Mum is dedicated to Glenda pro-actively and with such a hypersensitive way that I wonder if she ever takes a minute to sit and breathe and acknowledge herself!

The carer too, dedicated and a force of love and light. When I was pregnant with my daughter I led the sessions with a colleague of mine and could feel the dedication of this mother whose only relief from the anxiety and worry for her daughter seemed to be through the odd parties with friends and holidays away with her partner.

Then she would be back to her routine with her daughter. I remember thinking what if they (mum and carer) could get to the point where they did not have to go away to feel human or rejuvenated but find a way to be happy in themselves, connected; confident and healthy all the time. This in turn would have a powerful effect on Glenda.

These are only three little stories of parents/carers of a disabled child but there are so many more and there are so many more parents and carers who do not even realise they are! So many who struggle day in and day out without any help or time for recharging or simply having anyone to talk to.

The Power of the heart

According to Suzanne Scurlock-Durana a Craniosacral therapist practicing for many years in America many parents of children with additional and special needs have a hole in the backside of their heart. She says it is because these parents are so used to giving out unconditionally, that is the way they love, from the front of their hearts and why it is so open.

The way we love ourselves is from the back of the heart.

In these parents this space is empty.

So her advice is:

- to not identify those limiting beliefs you have about loving yourself and

- start to feel into the back of your heart. Breathe in here, this is a good start. Begin to communicate with his part of your body as a gentle way to begin caring for you.

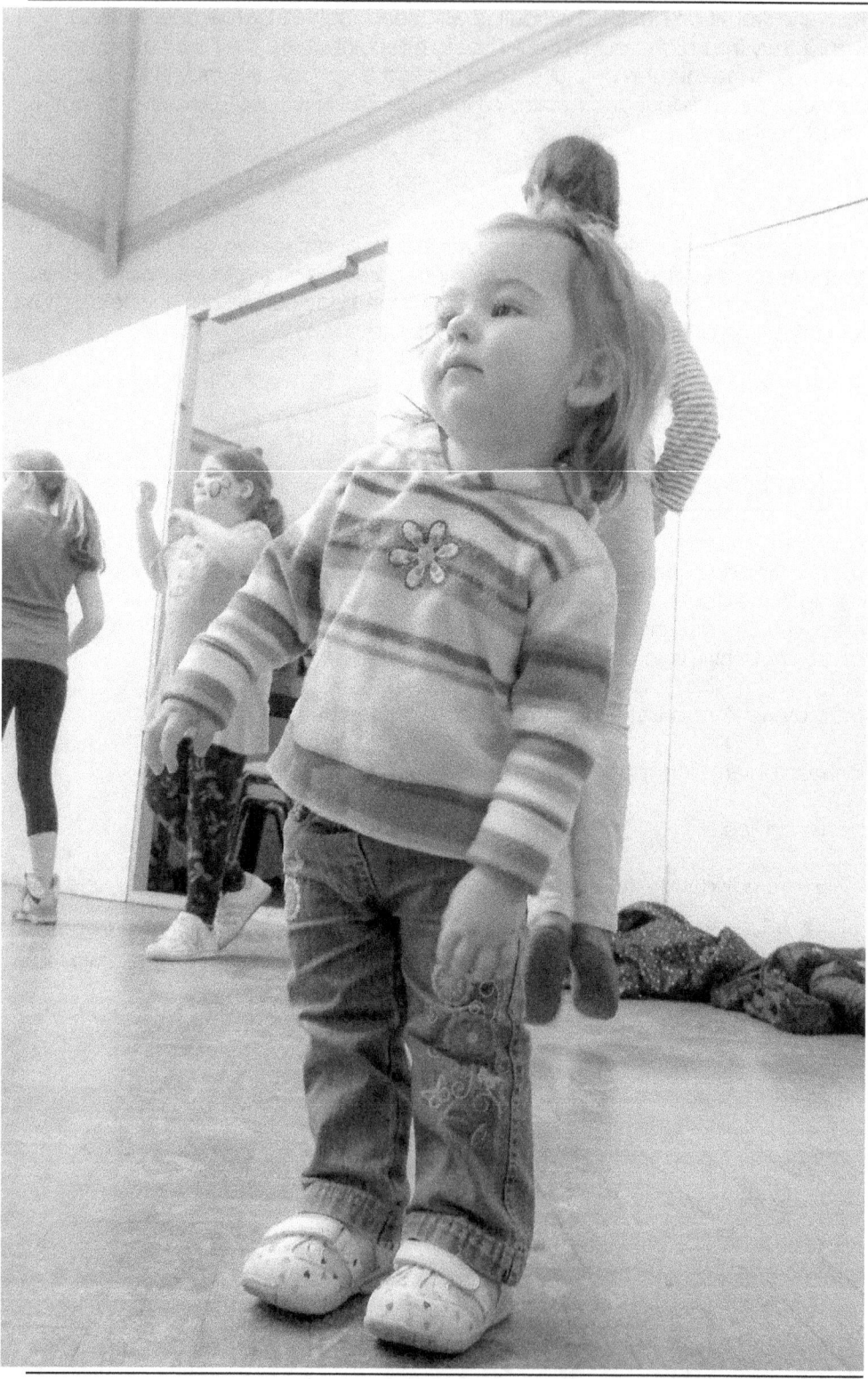

Karen Woodley - Movement Psychotherapy – RDMP

Healing Hands and Sensory Movement training programme

'Enlighten the lives of those you touch'

I offer a training course for Carers and those in the helping and healing professions that covers the person centred Approach to therapy and working with clients in this context as well as in depth coverage of the ways we can communicate. Essentially a movement based programme with simple daily life exercises and dances for health and well-being on all levels.

Healing Hands and Sensory Movement
Training Programme
'Enlighten the lives of those you touch'

Based in Creative Movement, Heart awareness and Affective Touch education for children and adults with additional needs, those with learning disabilities, the elderly and vulnerable groups who have difficulty in caring for themselves.

This training course has grown out of my research dissertation that found that it is only through an embodied relationship with our clients that we can make the most potent change. Having a vital awareness of your own bodily experience allows you to have access to the feeling of aliveness, memory, imagination, dreaming, play and all with a sense of agency in the world.

The course covers: Movement analysis (Rudolf Laban),
Attachment (John Bowlby), Love, the vital energy,
Attunement, the importance of play, Creativity (Rollo
May), the magic of music (Don Campbell), Laughter,
the importance of flow, the person centred model (Carl
Rogers) and Affective Touch development (R. Toro)

This programme is for health and well-being using dance and the affective human connection. The three building blocks that make this training so important are:

1. The body and its movement
2. Communication: disability or trauma
3. The voice of the Heart

The Approach is Holistic and Person Centred with a strong creative element where you will learn how to release negative energy held in the body and transform this into health. You will learn ways of working with different people and find out how to engage with the most vital and essential element of human kindness through your energy, through your body and through your desire to be a force of light and love in the world.

The training is for a minimum of four people each time and consists of 80 hours in total

- Workshop based sessions – 8 hours per day.

- Nonpresencial / homework – to be completed throughout the two week course

- Assessment will consist in student
  (1) leading a group in your community and
  (2) delivering a presentation on 'Sensory Movement and Communication' for a particular group.

- All materials for the course will be provided online

LOVE is what helps us to feel that at the deepest level we are seen, accepted and understood no matter your age, colour, race or religion! It is an energy that permeates everything and puts the real meaning back into life.

If we can re-learn to move with the sweet flow of human sweetness then our lives will have meaning! Through the universal language of music we are able to enter into our senses and life inside. Movement exploration, development and play help us to know and understand the world. And, nature helps us establish that sense of rhythm and timing.

From my experience for many years with learning disabilities, both children and adults, I have come to realise that if we stimulate all the senses then growth and change can happen. We learn, understand and feel in different ways the world around us but we all need to communicate in clear ways in order to be heard. For those who find this terribly difficult because of a disability or a trauma then it is vitally important to learn again.

Closing words

I hope you have enjoyed this book and have been inspired in some way through reading it into taking moments for self-care throughout your weeks.

I hope you have been moved a little step further into the wisdom and creativity of your own bodies and that you have gotten a few ideas of activities through music, movement and your own open hearts to use and communicate with.

I trust you will continue to explore the beautiful moments that give life shared with your clients/children/adults/ with love.

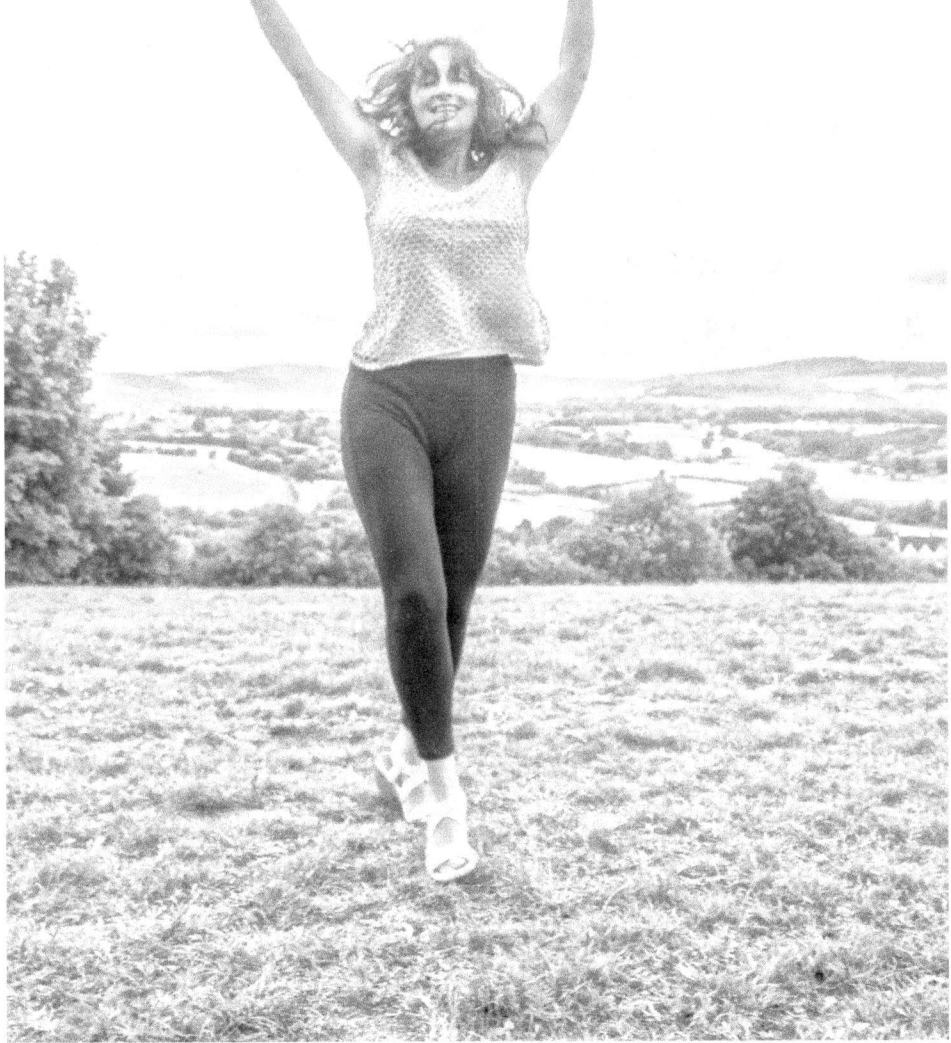

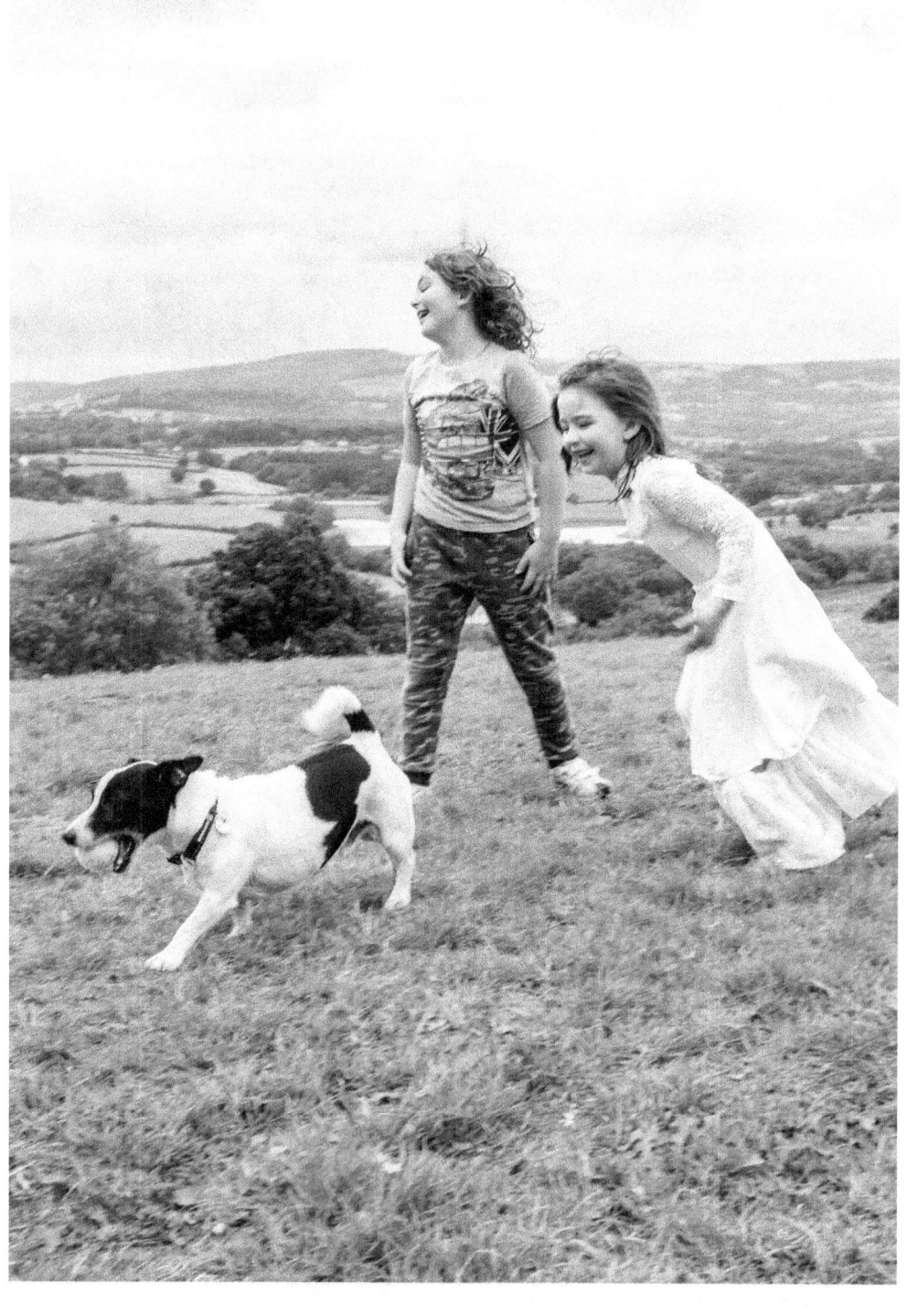

www.ingramcontent.com/pod-product-compliance
Lightning Source LLC
Chambersburg PA
CBHW070321290526
45791CB00003B/1201